MAYO CLINIC

Book of Alternative Medicine

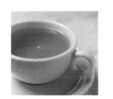 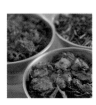 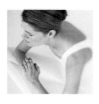

MAYO CLINIC

Medical Editor Brent Bauer, M.D.

Publisher Sara Gilliland

Editor in Chief, Books & Newsletters Christopher Frye

Managing Editor Karen Wallevand

Contributing Editors Richard Dietman, Kevin Kaufman

Creative Director Daniel Brevick

Art Directors S. Jay Koski, Paul Krause

Proofreaders Miranda Attlesey, Donna Hanson

Indexer Steve Rath

TIME INC. HOME ENTERTAINMENT

Publisher Richard Fraiman

Executive Director, Marketing Services Carol Pittard

Director, Retail & Special Sales Tom Mifsud

Marketing Director, Branded Business Swati Rao

Director, New Product Development Peter Harper

Financial Director Steven Sandonato

Assistant General Counsel Dasha Smith Dwin

Book Production Manager Suzanne Janso

Marketing Manager Victoria Alfonso

Design & Prepress Manager Anne-Michelle Gallero

Special thanks to: Bozena Bannett, Glenn Buonocore, Robert Marasco, Brooke McGuire, Jonathan Polsky, Chavaughn Raines, Mary Sarro-Waite, Ilene Schreider, Adriana Tierno

Published by Time Inc. Home Entertainment Books

Time Inc.
1271 Avenue of the Americas
New York, NY 10020

ISBN: 1-933405-92-9
  978-1933405-92-6

Library of Congress Control Number: 2006906801

First Edition

2 3 4 5 6 7 8 9 10

We welcome your comments and suggestions on *Mayo Clinic Book of Alternative Medicine*. Please write to us at TIHE Books, Attention: Book Editors, P. O. Box 11016, Des Moines, IA 50336-1016.

If you would like to order more copies of this book or any of our hardcover Collector's Edition books, please call 800-327-6388 (Monday through Friday, 7 a.m. to 8 p.m., or Saturday, 7 a.m. to 6 p.m. Central time).

For bulk sales to employers, member groups and health-related companies, contact Mayo Clinic Health Management Resources, 200 First St. S.W., Rochester, MN 55905, or send an e-mail to SpecialSalesMayoBooks@Mayo.edu.

Mayo Clinic Book of Alternative Medicine is intended to supplement the advice of your personal physician, whom you should consult regarding individual medical conditions. MAYO, MAYO CLINIC, MAYO CLINIC HEALTH INFORMATION and the Mayo triple-shield logo are marks of Mayo Foundation for Medical Education and Research.

Photo credits: Stock photography from Artville, BananaStock, Brand X Pictures, Comstock, Corbis, Creatas, Digital Stock, Digital Vision, EyeWire, Food Shapes, Image Ideas, Image Source, PhotoAlto, Photodisc, Pixtal, Rubberball and Stockbyte. The individuals pictured are models, and the photos are used for illustrative purposes only. There is no correlation between the individuals portrayed and the conditions or subjects being discussed. Photographs of Mayo specialists by Joseph Kane, Richard Madsen and Scott Dulla.

Jacket design by Daniel Brevick.

In this book we discuss a variety of products and practices. Our intent is for this information to serve as discussion points between the reader and his or her doctor. Because we say a therapy may be beneficial or we give it a "green light" does not mean we are endorsing any specific product.

Introduction

Most of us have grown up with a "fix-it" mentality when it comes to our health. We don't worry about it until something goes wrong — an illness develops — and then we go to the doctor to fix it. Those days are fading. As health care costs increase, greater responsibility is being — and will continue to be — placed on each of us to stay healthy and prevent disease.

It's in this environment — one in which Americans are seeking greater control of their health — that we've seen explosive growth in the field of complementary and alternative medicine. People are looking for more "natural" or "holistic" ways to maintain good health — not only their physical heath, but also their mental and spiritual health. At the same time, an increasing number of treatments once considered "on the fringe" are slowly being incorporated into conventional medicine.

We decided to write this book because we recognize the need for reliable and easy-to-understand information when it comes to complementary and alternative medicine. The purpose of *Mayo Clinic Book of Alternative Medicine* isn't only to inform you about various products and practices, but to guide you as to which appear to be of benefit and may help treat or prevent disease and which are of no benefit and could even be dangerous. The book can help lay the foundation for a truly holistic approach to health and wellness, however it's important that you include your doctor's advice in the decisions you make.

A note about the title of the book: As nontraditional products and practices gain greater acceptance as potential forms of healing, the terms used to describe them is evolving as well. Today, the term *integrative medicine* is often used to describe this evolving form of health care in which alternative therapies proved effective in scientific studies are being integrated with conventional care. But we're also aware that the latest changes in the medical field take time to filter down to the general public. *Alternative medicine* is still the term most commonly used to describe practices that aren't typically part of conventional medical care, or that are slowly being blended into conventional care.

That's why we decided to title this publication *Mayo Clinic Book of Alternative Medicine*. We feel it best describes to the reader what this book is about — nontraditional therapies to promote health and wellness. Inside, you'll find the latest information on how you might put some of these practices to work for you. By combining the best of complementary and conventional health care practices to meet your individual needs, you'll be practicing integrative medicine.

As you read through the pages ahead, here are a few important points to keep in mind. Some therapies don't fit neatly into a specific category. Reflexology, for instance, could go in either the hands-on therapies chapter or the chapter on energy therapies — it has components of both. Aromatherapy is another example. Some view it as a form of energy medicine, while others see it as a mind-body technique. We placed the therapies in the chapters we felt they fit best, but we recognize that many of them cross boundaries.

It's also important to understand that what's considered alternative or complementary today may be conventional tomorrow. In addition, using a particular therapy to treat one condition may be an accepted medical practice, but using it to treat another condition may not. A case in point is chiropractic care. There are numerous studies to back up the effectiveness of chiropractic therapy for treatment of low back pain. However, use of chiropractic techniques to treat high blood pressure would still be considered an alternative practice by many because there's not sufficient evidence that it's effective.

In the end, the names and classifications of the various therapies are going to become increasingly less important. What is important, is finding the best evidence-based products and practices that work with conventional medicine to improve your health — mind, body and spirit.

Brent A. Bauer

Brent Bauer, M.D.
Medical Editor

Table of Contents

Part 1

Today's New Medicine

Integrating alternative and conventional therapies

People who take an active role in their health care experience better health and improved healing. It's a common-sense concept gaining scientific roots.

As studies continue to reveal the important role the mind plays in healing and in fighting disease, a transformation is slowly taking place in hospitals and clinics across the country. Doctors, in partnership with their patients, are turning to practices once considered "alternative" as they attempt to treat the whole person — mind and spirit, as well as body.

In Part 1, we take a look at how alternative and complementary medicine is making inroads into conventional care, blending the best of nontraditional therapies with the best of high-tech medicine. We also discuss the important role you play in maintaining good health with the choices you make each day.

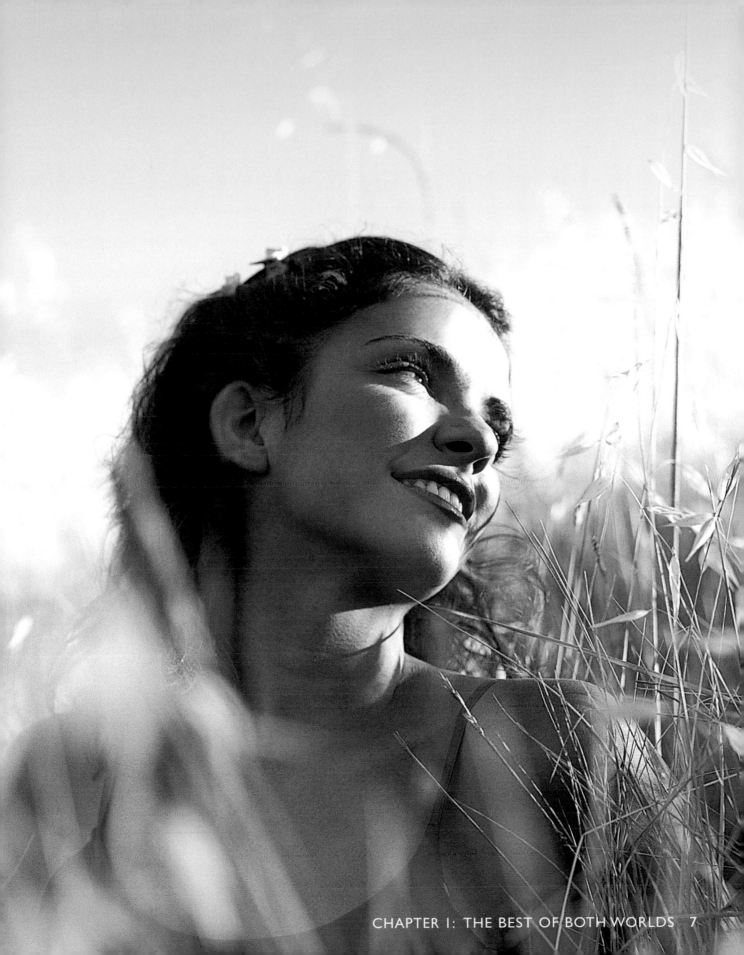

Chapter 1
The Best of Both Worlds

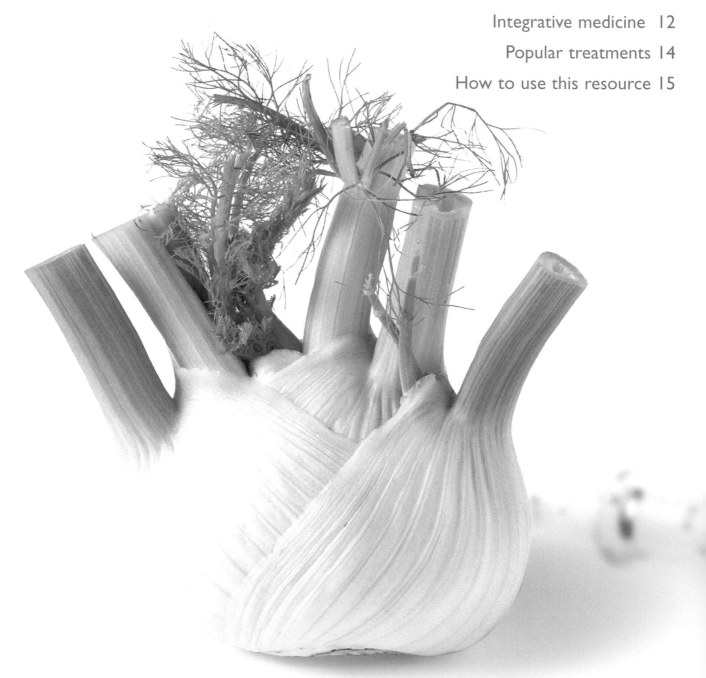

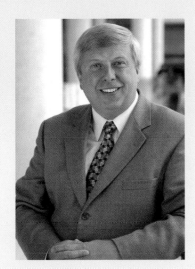

Brent Bauer, M.D.
Director, Complementary and Integrative Medicine Program

66 *Thanks to increased research during the past two decades, doctors are now better able to understand the role these 'alternative' therapies can play in helping treat and pre-vent disease.* 99

Kairos is a Greek word meaning "the critical time," and it's often thought of as the point in time when crisis and opportunity are equally balanced. Health care in the United States appears to be at a kairos moment — a combination of an aging population and wonderful, yet expensive, medical technology has resulted in sky-rocketing costs. At the same time, many people feel that medicine, in spite of its amazing advances, has become too technical and "cold."

In response to some of these changes, an opportunity has risen that may hold the promise of a new paradigm for better health. Called "unconventional" or "alter-native" medicine in the early '90s, then "complementary and alternative medi-cine" (CAM) until recently, new therapies and treatments are emerging to meet the needs of our physical, mental and spiritual health. Many of these therapies — such as massage therapy, herbal supplements and meditation — have been with us for a thousand years or more. What's "new" is the growing recognition that these practices may hold special value in meeting our health needs. Thanks to increased research during the past two decades, doctors are now better able to understand the role these alternative therapies can play in helping treat and pre-vent disease. This blending of the best of both worlds — conventional medicine and alternative medicine — is known as integrative medicine.

In this chapter and in future chapters, we share some of the exciting research tak-ing place at Mayo Clinic in the realm of integrative medicine. We also share some of the experience that our staff has had in working with thousands of individuals who have incorporated novel treatments into their health regimens. Unfortu-nately, there are pitfalls in this new realm — over-hyped products on the Internet that promise to cure every ill; unexpected side effects from common herbs such as St. John's wort; and individuals who have died because they made the mistake of believing that everything that's "natural" is safe.

Keep in mind, at this point in time, there's more that we don't know about inte-grative medicine than we do know. On the other hand, integrative medicine offers some wonderful opportunities to improve your health. Imagine having a "tool" that you can use the next time you're stuck in traffic and you feel your stress level rising, or a simple technique that may allow you to treat your high blood pressure with less medication. These are just a couple of the many ways this book can help you develop new strategies for improving your health.

In the end, we are all unique creations — what works for one person may not work for another. But that's part of the beauty of being able to select from a growing array of treatments and therapies. If meditation doesn't appeal to you or meet your needs, music therapy might. The important thing is not the spe-cific therapy or treatment, but making your health a top priority.

Alternative medicine

Whether it be herbs to battle a cold, meditation to help reduce high blood pressure or acupuncture to control pain, Americans are increasingly turning to health and healing practices outside of mainstream medicine.

As young and old alike seek greater control of their own health — either by choice or by circumstance — complementary and alternative therapies have become increasingly popular.

In the most recent government-funded survey, 36 percent of adults interviewed reported using some form of complementary or alternative medicine. That number rises to 62 percent when use of megavitamins and prayer are included.

Perhaps you just started using complementary or alternative therapies — or have become familiar with some of the products or practices. However, most of what we refer to as complementary and alternative medicine (CAM) isn't new. Many therapies have been in use for thousands of years.

What is new — or what has changed — is the attitude toward complementary and alternative medicine by the medical community. Even some of the most conservative health institutions have begun integrating therapies generally not part of mainstream medicine into their treatment programs.

Does this mean that all forms of complementary and alternative medicine are OK to use? No. Some carry significant risks and others simply don't work. It does indicate, though, that certain therapies do have merit and can aid in health and healing.

Complementary vs. alternative

The National Center for Complementary and Alternative Medicine, a division of the National Institutes of Health, defines complementary medicine as unconventional treatments used *in addition to* treatments by your doctor. An example is using tai chi in addition to a prescription medication to manage anxiety.

In contrast, alternative medicine includes treatments used *in place of* traditional medicine. This might include seeing a homeopath or naturopath instead of your regular doctor.

Among the general public, this distinction isn't as clear. Many people use the term *alternative medicine* as a catch all phrase to refer to both — therapies used in addition to conventional care and those used in place of it.

Guiding principles

Most products, practices and therapies are based around a few common principles:

- **Prevention.** One of the main philosophies of complemen-

tary and alternative medicine is to take preventive steps to promote good health.
- **Natural healing.** Your body has the ability to heal itself. The purpose of treatment is to encourage natural healing processes.
- **Active learning.** CAM practitioners see themselves as facilitators — teachers who offer guidance. You're the one who actually produces the healing.
- **'Holistic' care.** The focus is on treating the whole person — addressing physical, emotional, social and spiritual needs.

CAM figures

The most comprehensive and reliable findings to date on Americans' use of complementary and alternative medicine were released in 2004 by the National Center for Complementary and Alternative Medicine (NCCAM) and the National Center for Health Statistics (NCHS).

The figures came from the NCHS's National Health Interview Survey, in which tens of thousands of Americans are interviewed annually about their health. The focus of one year's survey was on use of complementary and alternative medicine.

Take 10

Just how much do you know about alternative and complementary medicine? Take this short quiz and see how you do.

1. **The most commonly used alternative and complementary therapy in the United States is:**
   a) prayer
   b) meditation
   c) herbal supplements
   d) chiropractic care

2. **The percentage of American adults who use some form of complementary or alternative medicine is:**
   a) 27%
   b) 49%
   c) 62%
   d) 84%

3. **Women are more likely to use complementary and alternative therapies than are men:**
   a) true
   b) false

4. **The most common condition for which people turn to complementary and alternative medicine is:**
   a) anxiety
   b) arthritis
   c) back pain
   d) common cold

5. **The most common reason people give for using a complementary or alternative therapy is:**
   a) thought it would be interesting to try
   b) wanted to try something in addition to conventional treatments
   c) thought conventional treatments wouldn't help
   d) their doctor suggested they try it

6. **Approximately how much money is spent yearly on complementary and alternative therapies?**
   a) $36 million to $47 million
   b) $360 million to $470 million
   c) $3.6 billion to $4.7 billion
   d) $36 billion to $47 billion

7. **Some forms of complementary and alternative medicine have been practiced for more than 1,000 years:**
   a) true
   b) false

8. **'Integrative medicine' refers to:**
   a) healing of mind, body and spirit
   b) whole-body treatment vs. symptoms-based care
   c) combining complementary and alternative therapies with conventional medicine
   d) all of the above

9. **Diet and exercise are the foundation of optimal health:**
   a) true
   b) false

10. **Studies don't support a correlation between mental and physical health:**
    a) true
    b) false

Answers: 1. a, 2. c, 3. a, 4. c, 5. b, 6. d, 7. a, 8. d, 9. a, 10. b

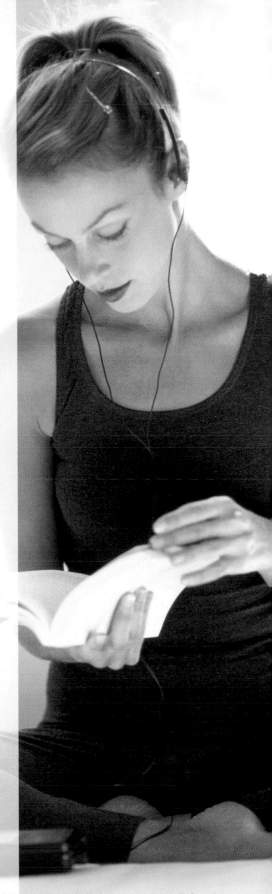

Integrative medicine

The term *integrative medicine* may be new to you. However, you already may be experiencing integrative medicine and you just aren't aware of it.

Medicine of the future

Integrative medicine is a fairly new concept that describes a growing movement taking place in many health care institutions — integrating complementary and alternative therapies with conventional medicine.

The goal of integrative medicine is to treat the whole person — mind, body and spirit — not just the disease. This is done by combining the best of today's high-tech medicine with the best of nontraditional practices — therapies that have some high-quality evidence to support their use.

Why the interest in doing so? Not that long ago, scientists viewed the connection between mind and body with skepticism. But research continues to unveil the complex biology of how the two are intertwined, and how treating the mind and spirit can help to heal the body.

This is why in addition to a prescription medication to treat your migraines your doctor may also recommend biofeedback training to reduce stress.

It's also clear that interest in complementary and alternative medicine isn't a passing fad. As more individuals turn to unconventional treatments, doctors are all too aware of the need for quality research to determine their safety and effectiveness.

Integrative Medicine at Mayo Clinic

Mayo Clinic's Complementary and Integrative Medicine Consult Service was developed in 2001 to address interest by patients in products and practices not typically part of conventional medical care — treatments such as meditation, massage therapy, and use of herbs and other dietary supplements. Specialty-trained doctors and other health professionals within the consultation service work with patients, and their doctors, to provide information on nontraditional therapies and to encourage healing and wellness through a variety of channels.

The treatments promoted through the complementary and integrative medicine program aren't substitutes for conventional medical care. They're used in concert with medical treatment to help alleviate stress, reduce pain and anxiety, manage symptoms, maintain strength and flexibility, and promote a sense of well-being.

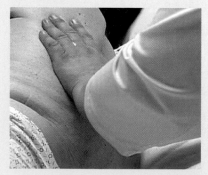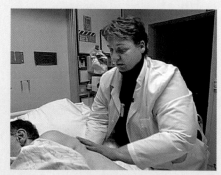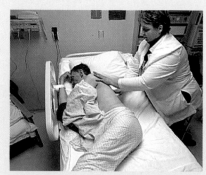

A Mayo Clinic massage therapist performs massage therapy after cardiovascular surgery to reduce pain and anxiety. On the opposite page, Mayo researchers study ancient texts in search of lost medicinal therapies.

Turning ideas into treatments

An important part of the mission of Mayo Clinic's Complementary and Integrative Medicine Program is to learn more about unconventional products and practices to determine if they can play a role in health and healing.

Presently, the program is involved in more than 25 studies. Here are a few examples:

Massage therapy

Does your anxiety level and state of mind after cardiovascular surgery affect your recovery? Early indications are, the answer is "yes."

Mayo researchers are just concluding a study in which individuals received massage therapy after cardiovascular surgery. Initial results indicate the therapy helped decrease pain and anxiety after surgery.

'Ambience' therapy

Researchers are studying whether playing music in hospital rooms — specifically, music mixed with sounds of nature — can reduce side effects and speed recovery after cardiovascular surgery.

The music, known as "ambience" therapy, was produced by Chip Davis from the group Mannheim Steamroller.

Ginseng

A common problem for individuals undergoing treatment for cancer is fatigue that typically accompanies chemotherapy or radiation therapy. Mayo researchers in the Integrative Medicine Program are evaluating the effects of the herb ginseng to determine if it can help offset cancer-related fatigue.

Ginkgo

Another potential side effect of cancer treatment is what's referred to as "chemobrain" — a slowing of mental functioning that sometimes develops months after chemotherapy treatment. This phenomenon is thought to be related to oxidative stress on cells from the drug therapy.

To combat chemobrain, some people take antioxidative supplements, such as ginkgo. The question is, do the supplements interfere with the effectiveness of cancer treatment? Mayo researchers hope to find out.

Valerian

The herb valerian is the focus of yet another cancer-related study. Valerian is taken to help induce sleep. Researchers want to find out if it works and if it can promote sleep in cancer patients who often experience difficulty sleeping while undergoing treatment.

Yoga

An important component of yoga is its methodic breathing, what's referred to as "paced respirations." This form of breathing is used to help alleviate stress and anxiety. Can it also help relieve hot flashes? Researchers are checking into it.

Participants in the study are breast cancer survivors who have limited treatment options for hot flashes because hormone therapy generally isn't advised for this group. If effective, the treatment should also work in women who don't have cancer.

Plant compounds

Mayo researchers are studying a 400-year-old catalogue of plants (botanicals) used by ancient healers of the South Pacific. The catalogue was written by German-Dutch naturalist Georg Eberhard Rumphius. Researchers are hoping to resurrect lost healing knowledge from ancient texts. The Dutch text has lead to further exploration of a series of compounds that may hold promise as future therapies.

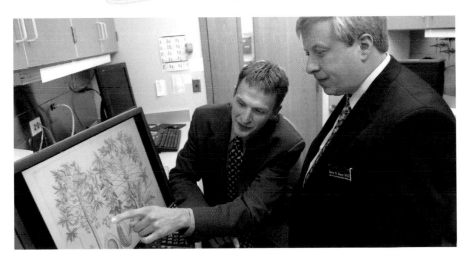

Popular treatments

The National Center for Complementary and Alternative Medicine and the National Center for Health Statistics are continuing their efforts to learn more about why people use complementary and alternative therapies and which are the most popular. Here's what their most recent survey found:

Reasons for use

The survey asked participants to select from five reasons why they use complementary and alternative therapies. They could select more than one reason.

Results indicated that most people use conventional and alternative medicine (CAM) to supplement the care they receive from their doctor, rather than in place of conventional treatment.

Therapies used most often

The most commonly used complementary and alternative therapy is prayer. This includes praying for your own health and having others pray for your health.

Following prayer is use of "natural products." In this specific survey, natural products included herbs and other plant-based products, as well as animal-based dietary products. It didn't include the use of vitamins and minerals.

Natural products used most often

About one in five people surveyed use supplements (natural products) to enhance their health. The product most commonly used is the herb echinacea, followed by the herbs ginseng and ginkgo.

The chart on page 15 lists the most popular natural products. The percentage represents the rate of use among adults who use dietary supplements.

Health conditions prompting use

People use complementary and alternative practices for a wide array of diseases and conditions.

Americans most often turn to unconventional therapies to treat or prevent muscle- or skeletal-related conditions that produce chronic or recurrent pain.

Most Common Reasons

Reason	Percentage who gave it
1. Thought combining CAM with conventional medicine would help	54.9%
2. Thought it would be interesting to try	50.1%
3. Thought conventional medicine would not help	27.7%
4. A conventional medicine professional suggested it	25.8%
5. Conventional medicine too expensive	13.2%

Source: National Center for Health Statistics, 2004

Most Common Therapies

Type of therapy	Percentage who use it
1. Prayer for own health	43.0%
2. Others' prayer for your health	24.4%
3. Natural products*	18.9%
4. Deep-breathing exercises	11.6%
5. Prayer group participation for own health	9.6%
6. Meditation	7.6%
7. Chiropractic care	7.5%
8. Yoga	5.1%
9. Massage	5.0%
10. Diet-based therapies	3.5%

*This figure doesn't include use of megavitamins or minerals

How to use this resource

Doctors and other staff in the Mayo Clinic Complementary and Integrative Medicine Program developed this publication to provide you straightforward information about various therapies being used and what's known about them.

With each treatment, we discuss the latest research, the safety and effectiveness of the product or practice, and any potential risks, should you decide to try it.

We also talk about the importance of good lifestyle habits to ensure you get the most out of the efforts you're making to improve your health. *Mayo Clinic Book of Alternative Medicine* is a personal health guide that can help you achieve great health and fully enjoy life.

About the lights

A special feature of this book — which you'll find in upcoming pages — is our stoplight. Its purpose is to give you an at-a-glance overview as to how you should proceed with the therapy being discussed.

A shining red light means not to use the treatment or to use it very carefully and only under a doctor's close supervision. A therapy is given a red light when studies have found it to be unsafe or have found its risks far outweigh any benefits it may provide.

A shining yellow light means to use the therapy with caution. A treatment is given a yellow light when studies show it may be of benefit but that it also carries some risks. Therapies that have not been fully studied to determine their safety and effectiveness are also given a yellow light. In addition, a treatment may be given a yellow light if it's considered safe, but studies haven't found it to provide any benefit.

A shining green light means the therapy is generally safe for most people to use, and studies show it to be effective. (If you have a specific health condition, a therapy given a green light may not be appropriate for you.) Even when a green light is present, it's still important that you discuss the treatment with your doctor and use it appropriately.

Most Common Natural Products

Name of product	Percentage who use it
1. Echinacea	40.3%
2. Ginseng	24.1%
3. Ginkgo biloba	21.1%
4. Garlic supplements	19.9%
5. Glucosamine	14.9%
6. St. John's wort	12.0%
7. Peppermint	11.8%
8. Fish oil/omega-3 fatty acids	11.7%
9. Ginger supplements	10.5%
10. Soy supplements	9.4%

Most Common Conditions

Condition	Percentage who cited it
1. Back pain	16.8%
2. Head cold	9.5%
3. Neck pain	6.6%
4. Joint pain	4.9%
5. Arthritis	4.9%
6. Anxiety/depression	4.5%
7. Stomach upset	3.7%
8. Headache	3.1%
9. Recurring pain	2.4%
10. Insomnia	2.2%

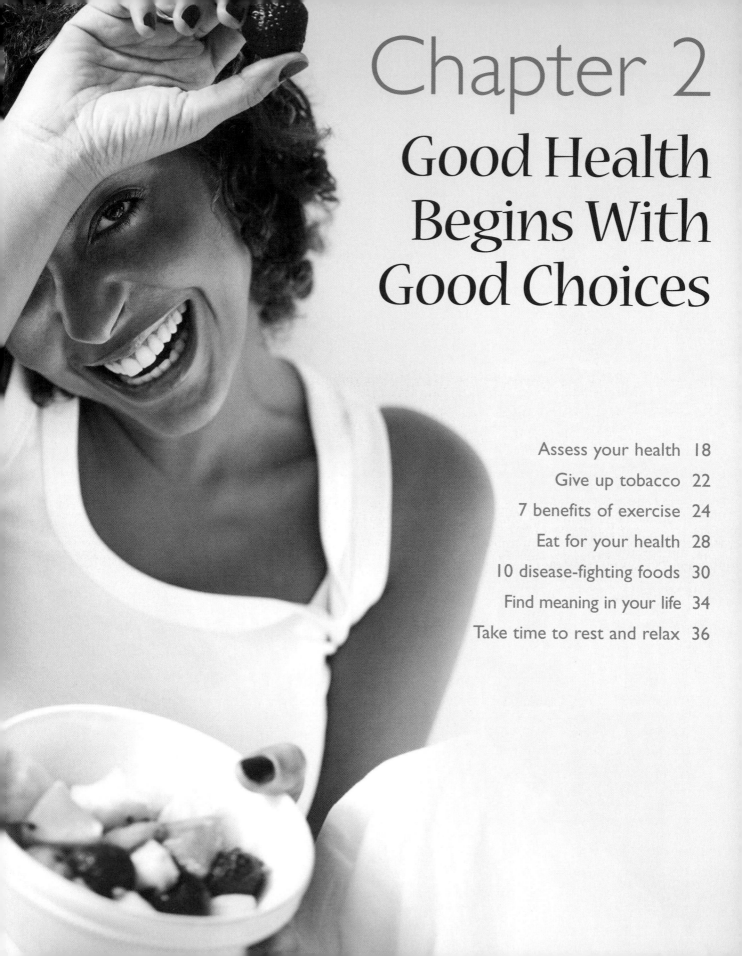

Chapter 2

Good Health Begins With Good Choices

A visit with Dr. Paul Limburg

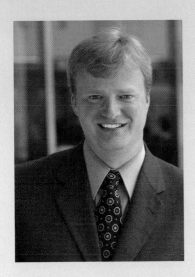

Paul Limburg, M.D., M.P.H.
Gastroenterology

“ The fact is, if you spend most of your day lying on the couch and eating potato chips, taking a supplement to help you lose weight or practicing techniques to boost your immune system likely isn't going to do you much good. ”

Congratulations! By reading this chapter, you've taken the first step in adopting a healthier lifestyle. And why is lifestyle important in a book about alternative medicine? The fact is, if you spend most of your day lying on the couch and eating potato chips, taking a supplement to help you lose weight or practicing techniques to boost your immune system likely isn't going to do you much good. To fend off disease and achieve better health, you need to take care of yourself.

Let's face it — most people, including doctors, find countless excuses for why they can't change their unhealthy behaviors. Change is difficult for everyone. However, adopting healthier habits doesn't have to be painful. And once you're able to learn new habits, the quality of your life can improve dramatically.

In the pages that follow, we focus on five key areas where good lifestyle choices have been shown to reduce the development of — or consequences related to — several common medical conditions, including cardiovascular disease, cancer and diabetes. These five areas are tobacco use, diet (including alcohol consumption), weight control, exercise and stress management. Clearly, trying to address all of these issues at once would be difficult. Therefore, we've included an easy-to-use checklist in the first few pages that can help you determine which of these factors are most relevant to your own personal health. We also provide recommendations for how to improve unhealthy habits.

As you begin, or continue, to think about making healthier lifestyle choices, keep in mind that the best results will come from long-term, rather than short-term, changes — a useful analogy might be to consider the process a marathon, not a sprint. What does this mean? First, start by finding an appropriate balance between positive lifestyle changes and family, job, social and other responsibilities. Don't let competing priorities get in the way of good health. Second, define milestones to help you monitor your progress. Reward yourself when you achieve your goals so that productive changes are reinforced. Just as importantly, challenge yourself when you fall short so that potential obstacles can be identified and avoided. Third, don't give up if your first attempt isn't successful. Learn from your effort, make necessary adjustments and try again, perhaps using an alternative approach. Last, involve people around you who might derive benefits from the healthy lifestyle habits you're trying to develop. Making changes can be easier if relatives, friends or colleagues are fully supportive.

In later chapters, we show you how complementary and alternative therapies can provide new opportunities to help you meet your wellness goals.

Assess your health

Over the next four pages we ask a few basic questions about your health to help you evaluate your lifestyle habits and determine your health risks.

If you breeze through the questions, you're probably already making good choices. If not, the questions should point to changes you can make for improvements.

The healthier you are, the greater the chances that other efforts you make to fight disease and stay healthy — including the use of complementary and alternative therapies — will be beneficial.

Do you use tobacco?

Do you smoke or use spit tobacco?

Yes _____ Tobacco use is a tough habit to break, but stopping could be the single most important health change you make. See pages 22-23 for tips on how to give up tobacco.

No _____ Go to the next question.

Basic tobacco quit plan

1. List five reasons for quitting.
2. Set a quit date.
3. Get rid of all tobacco on your quit date.
4. Get support from family, friends and co-workers.
5. Find alternatives to the habit, such as nicotine replacement products and lifestyle changes.

Tobacco facts

More than 400,000 Americans die of tobacco-related illnesses each year. If you smoke a pack of cigarettes a day and you quit, you'll save about $1,500 a year.

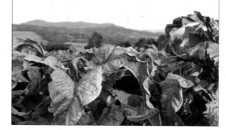

Do you get enough exercise?

How many minutes a week do you spend doing moderate or vigorous physical activities? Check the time that comes closest. (Note: For most people, moderate or vigorous activities include brisk walking, dancing, biking, swimming and running).

0 to 30 minutes _____
You need to be more physically active. If there are health reasons why you're not more active, ask your doctor about an exercise plan that's right for you.

30 to 90 minutes _____
You're off to a good start! Try to gradually increase the amount of time you exercise.

90 to 120 minutes _____
You're well on your way to being physically fit. If you're doing vigorous activity, you've reached a reasonable goal when you're doing 90 minutes or more a week.

120 minutes or more _____
You're an active person and probably at a good level of fitness. If weight loss is part of your plan, you may need at least 200 minutes a week of moderate physical activity.

Basic activity plan

1. Aim to do something nearly every day of the week.
2. Set a goal of a specific number of minutes or steps a week.
3. Keep a log to help remind you and track your progress.
4. Recruit a friend or family member to keep you company.
5. Build up slowly, but steadily.
   If you're having difficulty or not feeling well while doing physical activities, see your doctor.

Fitness fact

More than 60 percent of American adults aren't physically active on a regular basis, and 25 percent aren't active at all. Even a modest walking program (see page 27) can improve your heart health, reduce stress and give you extra energy to do the things you enjoy.

How's your weight?

Determine your body mass index (BMI) and your waist circumference to see if you're in the healthy weight zone. To do this, you'll need a bathroom scale and a tape measure.

To determine your BMI use the handy BMI chart and write your BMI here. _____

Next, measure the narrowest part of your abdomen to determine your waist circumference and write the number here.

_____

If your BMI is less than 18.5, talk with your doctor. You may be at risk of health conditions associated with a low body weight.

If your BMI is within the range of 19 to 24, you're at a healthy weight.

If your BMI is 25 or greater, consider losing some weight.

As for your waist circumference, a healthy goal is 40 inches or less if you're a man and 35 inches or less if you're a woman.

Basic weight-loss plan

1. Set a weight-loss goal of 1 to 2 pounds a week.
2. Eat five or more servings of fruits and vegetables daily.
3. Work with your health care provider to develop an exercise plan.
4. Gradually increase the time you spend on physical activity to at least 30 minutes a day.
5. Recruit a friend or family member for support.

Body mass index (BMI)

You can determine your body mass index (BMI) by finding your height and weight on this chart. A BMI of 18.5 to 24.9 is considered the healthiest. People with a BMI under 18.5 are considered underweight. People with a BMI between 25 and 29.9 are considered overweight. People with a BMI of 30 or greater are considered obese.

BMI	Healthy		Overweight					Obese				
	19	24	25	26	27	28	29	30	35	40	45	50
Height					Weight in pounds							
4'10"	91	115	119	124	129	134	138	143	167	191	215	239
4'11"	94	119	124	128	133	138	143	148	173	198	222	247
5'0"	97	123	128	133	138	143	148	153	179	204	230	255
5'1"	100	127	132	137	143	148	153	158	185	211	238	264
5'2"	104	131	136	142	147	153	158	164	191	218	246	273
5'3"	107	135	141	146	152	158	163	169	197	225	254	282
5'4"	110	140	145	151	157	163	169	174	204	232	262	291
5'5"	114	144	150	156	162	168	174	180	210	240	270	300
5'6"	118	148	155	161	167	173	179	186	216	247	278	309
5'7"	121	153	159	166	172	178	185	191	223	255	287	319
5'8"	125	158	164	171	177	184	190	197	230	262	295	328
5'9"	128	162	169	176	182	189	196	203	236	270	304	338
5'10"	132	167	174	181	188	195	202	209	243	278	313	348
5'11"	136	172	179	186	193	200	208	215	250	286	322	358
6'0"	140	177	184	191	199	206	213	221	258	294	331	368
6'1"	144	182	189	197	204	212	219	227	265	302	340	378
6'2"	148	186	194	202	210	218	225	233	272	311	350	389
6'3"	152	192	200	208	216	224	232	240	279	319	359	399
6'4"	156	197	205	213	221	230	238	246	287	328	369	410

Note: Asians with a BMI of 23 or higher may have an increased risk of health problems.
Source: National Institutes of Health, 1998

Weight fact

More than two-thirds of all Americans are overweight. Being overweight increases your risk of diabetes, arthritis, heart disease, cancer and sleep disorders. Slow, steady weight loss is the best way to get to a healthy weight.

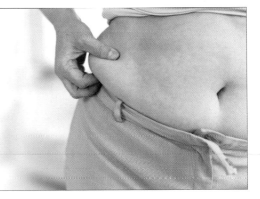

Is your diet healthy?

How many servings of:
Fruits do you eat each day?

———

Vegetables do you eat each day?

———

Total = ———

If your total is five or greater, you're doing great. Keep up the good work. If not, look for ways to add more fruits and vegetables to your diet.

Basic healthy-eating plan

1. Add one additional fruit or vegetable serving each week until you're getting five or more servings most days.
2. Look for ways to reduce fat in your diet and increase whole grains.
3. Eat three healthy meals — including breakfast — every day.
4. Try at least one new healthy recipe each week.

Nutrition fact

Eating the right foods can prevent disease. Fiber — found in fruits, vegetables and whole grains — may lower your risk of diabetes. Vitamins and other nutrients in fresh or frozen fruits and vegetables may reduce your risk of some cancers and cardiovascular disease. Replacing butter, lard and other solid fats with healthier fats like olive, canola and peanut oils can help lower your risk of heart disease.

Alcohol and your health

Studies suggest that drinking moderate amounts of alcohol may increase levels of protective high-density lipoprotein (HDL or "good") cholesterol and reduce the risk of cardiovascular disease. But it's important not to forget the risks of alcohol.

Even small amounts of alcohol can slow brain activity, affecting alertness, coordination and reaction time. Alcohol also can interfere with sleep and sexual function, induce headaches, and contribute to heartburn. Heavy drinking can increase risk of death from all causes.

Drinking alcohol can also increase blood triglycerides and blood pressure and interfere with the effectiveness of some blood pressure medications. And the American Cancer Society links alcohol use with increased risk of cancers of the breast, liver, mouth, throat and esophagus.

Until more is known about the effects of alcohol on overall health, if you don't drink don't start. If you do drink, use moderation. Moderation equates to one alcoholic drink a day for nonpregnant women and anyone age 65 or older. For men under age 65, moderation is no more than two drinks a day. Pregnant women shouldn't drink any alcohol.

One drink equals 5 ounces of wine, 12 ounces of beer or 1.5 ounces of 80-proof liquor.

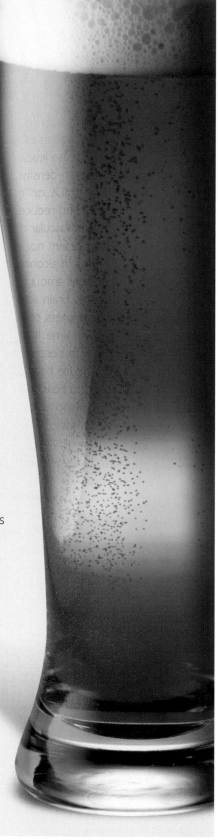

How's your mood?

For at least the past two weeks, have you persistently felt anxious, down or depressed?

Yes _____ Consider mentioning this to your doctor.

No _____ Go to the next question.

For at least the past two weeks, have you had little interest or pleasure in doing things?

Yes _____ Consider mentioning this to your doctor.

No _____

Basic stress management plan

1. Exercise at least 30 minutes most days of the week to help relieve stress and anxiety.
2. Aim for an average of eight hours of sleep each night.
3. Stay connected with family and friends.
4. Consider starting a meditation program (see page 90).

Mood fact

Stress and a depressed mood can increase your risk of heart disease, and they can intensify physical symptoms, such as pain.

What are your biggest health threats?

Why is it important to know what threatens your health? It's not to scare you, but rather to help guide you in the choices you make regarding your health and safety. The news is full of stories about avian flu, terrorism, floods and hurricanes. These global issues are important, but they may not be the greatest threat to your health. What should you work hardest to avoid? Check out the biggest risks to your health and well-being.

RANK	Causes of Most "Lost Productive Years of Life"	Most Common Causes of Death in All Ages	Causes of Death in Infants	Causes of Death in Children 1-14	Causes of Death in Young Adults 15-44	Causes of Death in Adults 45-64	Causes of Death in Adults 65 and older
Top 5 Leading Causes of Death and Lost Productive Years in the United States							
1	Cancer 23%	Heart Disease	Complications of Birth (Perinatal Death)	Motor Vehicle Accidents	Motor Vehicle Accidents	Cancer	Heart Disease
2	Heart Disease 22%	Cancer	Birth Defects	Other Accidents	Cancer	Heart Disease	Cancer
3	Motor Vehicle Accidents 5%	Stroke	Sudden Infant Death Syndrome (SIDS)	Cancer	Other Accidents	Diabetes	Stroke
4	Stroke 5%	Chronic Lung Disease	Accidents	Birth Defects	Heart Disease	Stroke	Lung Disease
5	Chronic Lung Disease 4%	Diabetes	Lung Disease	Homicide	Suicide	Lung Disease	Alzheimer's Disease

Modified from Centers for Disease Control and Prevention and National Center for Health Statistics Information, 2002-2003

Give up tobacco

A key strategy for living a longer, healthier life comes as no surprise — don't smoke. If you're a smoker, you're simply more likely to die prematurely. Smoking can take more than 10 years off your life.

But there's good news. Quitting now means health benefits start in just minutes, and your risk of heart disease is cut in half in as little as a year.

Strategies to help you quit

Success at quitting smoking is the result of planning and commitment, not luck. Develop a plan for how you'll cope with symptoms of nicotine withdrawal and how you'll survive urges to smoke.

Using more than one strategy to stop smoking might increase your chances of quitting successfully.

- **Medication.** Medication helps reduce cravings and eases withdrawal symptoms until the worst effects are over. You have many options — both prescription and over-the-counter products.
- **Cold turkey.** This is a sudden, decisive break from cigarettes. You stop smoking completely with little or no reduction beforehand. If you quit cold turkey, you're likely to experience symptoms of withdrawal, like nearly every-

one else who quits smoking. Some form of medication is usually recommended.

- **Taper down.** With this approach you gradually reduce the number of cigarettes you smoke until you don't smoke any at all. Medication is recommended with this approach as well.
- **Group support.** Whether it's an in-person support group, over the phone or online, seek the support of others who are trying to stop smoking.
- **Individual counseling.** This includes one-on-one contact with a trusted doctor, psychologist, nurse or counselor. This gives you a forum to discuss the barriers you have to quitting and, once you stop smoking, the urges you may have to light up again.
- **Telephone quitlines.** Counseling over the telephone has become an increasingly popular and accessible way for people to receive help for their smoking. Telephone counseling allows participants to receive an intensive intervention that's almost identical to face-to-face consultation.
- **Buddy system.** Ask a non-smoking friend or family member to be available when you experience tough times or when you have a reason to celebrate.

Keep in mind that what works for some people won't work for others. Talk with your doctor about your options and what might work best for you.

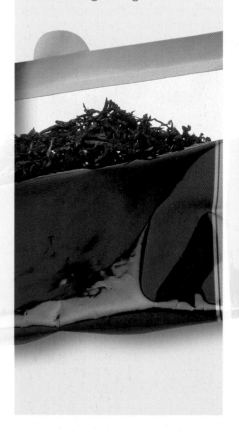

No kidding

Tobacco is tobacco. One form isn't any less dangerous than another. Using other types of tobacco products or cigarette alternatives — light cigarettes, cigars, pipes, snuff and chewing tobacco — can endanger your health just as much as regular cigarettes.

Medications to help you quit

Product	Pros	Cons	Cautions
Nicotine patch	Easy to use. Provides steady release of nicotine.	Can't quickly adjust amount to respond to craving. May cause skin irritation.	May not be appropriate if you have certain skin conditions.
Nicotine gum	Can chew it as often as needed. Keeps your mouth busy.	May cause gum or mouth soreness. May cause nausea or hiccups if chewed too fast.	As with all forms of nicotine replacement, don't use it while smoking.
Nicotine lozenges	Quickly satisfy cravings. Can use as needed.	May cause nausea, heartburn or hiccups.	Don't chew or swallow whole.
Nicotine inhaler	Keeps your hands and mouth busy. You control the dose.	May cause coughing and mouth or throat irritation.	May not be appropriate if you have lung disease, such as asthma.
Nicotine nasal spray	Reaches bloodstream quickly and works faster than other products.	May cause nasal, sinus and throat irritation, watery eyes and sneezing.	Not recommended for people with a nasal or sinus condition, allergies or asthma.
Bupropion (Zyban)	Easy-to-use pill. Doesn't contain nicotine.	Can cause insomnia and dry mouth.	Not appropriate for people with seizures or eating disorders, who already take medication containing bupropion, or who take an MAOI antidepressant.
Varenicline (Chantix)	Eases withdrawal symptoms. Blocks effects of nicotine if you resume smoking.	May cause stomach upset, headache and insomnia.	People with kidney disease may not be able to take it.

Beyond the basics

Two alternative therapies people use to help them quit smoking are hypnosis (see page 89) and acupuncture (see page 106). While there isn't strong evidence that either is highly effective for smoking cessation, they're relatively safe. If you think they can help you quit, it might be worth it to give one or both a try.

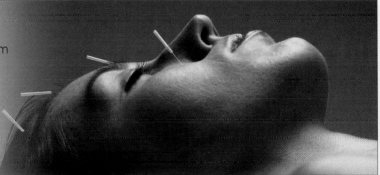

7 benefits of exercise

Imagine that a new wonder formula has been created. It will prevent illness and disease, help you lose weight, fight stress and put you in a better mood. It can also slow the aging process and make you feel younger.

Now imagine that this formula doesn't cost a penny and you can take it several times a day or just once a day and still see results.

Sounds appealing, doesn't it? Well, this miracle formula is already available. It's called exercise. Regular, old-fashioned exercise is one of the most important things you can do to fight disease and enjoy life. The merits of exercise — ranging from preventing chronic diseases to boosting your confidence — are hard to ignore.

Here are seven ways exercise can have a positive impact on your health.

1. Strengthens your cardiovascular and respiratory systems

Exercise reduces the buildup of harmful deposits (plaques) in your arteries by increasing the concentration of high-density lipoprotein (HDL or "good") cholesterol in your blood.

Exercise also strengthens your heart so that it can pump blood more efficiently. And it reduces the risk of developing high blood pressure, even if you're already at increased risk of it.

Plus, exercise benefits your respiratory system by promoting rhythmic, deep breathing.

2. Keeps bones and muscles strong

Physical activity is likely the single most important factor in maintaining bone density. It

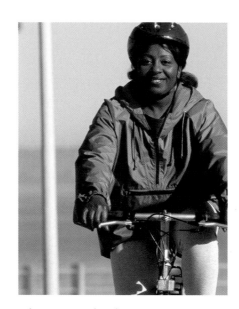

plays several roles in preventing and treating osteoporosis, perhaps most importantly by strengthening your bones.

3. Helps manage weight

Coupled with a healthy diet, exercise can help people lose weight, improving diseases and conditions associated with being overweight.

4. Prevents and manages diabetes

Regular exercise and a healthy diet reduce your risk of developing type 2 diabetes and can help control diabetes in individuals who already have it. Mild to moderate exercise helps the hormone insulin work better, lowering blood sugar levels.

5. Eases stress, depression and pain

Exercise fights stress, depression and pain by activating certain neurotransmitters — chemicals used by your nerve cells to communicate with one another.

These chemicals provide feelings of well-being that are associated with avoiding depression. They help you to relax and they provide "natural" pain relief.

6. Reduces your risk of certain cancers

Regular exercise may help lower the risk of cancers of the colon, breast, prostate, uterine lining (endometrium) and perhaps others.

Although it hasn't been proved, researchers think that exercise also helps combat colon cancer by causing digested food to move through the colon more quickly.

7. Helps you sleep better

Moderate exercise at least three hours before bedtime can help you relax and sleep better at night. A good night's sleep helps maintain your physical and mental health.

How fit are you?

Fitness isn't about how you look. It's about your health. Small increases in your fitness level can make a big difference in your overall well-being. Answer these questions.

Do you have enough energy to do the things you like to do?
① Rarely or never
② Sometimes
③ Always or most of the time

Do you have enough stamina and strength to carry out the daily tasks of your life?
① Rarely or never
② Sometimes
③ Always or most of the time

Can you walk a mile without feeling winded or fatigued?
① No
② Sometimes
③ Yes

Can you climb two flights of stairs without feeling winded or fatigued?
① No
② Sometimes
③ Yes

Can you do at least five push-ups before you need to stop for a rest?
① No
② Sometimes
③ Yes

Are you flexible enough to touch your toes while standing?
① No
② Sometimes
③ Yes

Can you carry on a conversation while doing light to moderate activities, such as brisk walking?
① No
② Sometimes
③ Yes

About how many days a week do you spend doing at least 30 minutes of moderately vigorous activity, such as walking briskly or raking leaves?
① Two days or less
② Three or four days
③ Five to seven days

About how many days a week do you spend doing at least 20 minutes of vigorous activity, such as jogging, participating in an aerobics dance class or playing singles tennis?
① None
② One to three
③ Four or more

About how many minutes do you walk during the day, including walking the dog, doing chores around the house, walking from your car to the office or store, or doing errands at work?
① Less than 30 minutes
② 30 to 60 minutes
③ More than 60 minutes

How did you score?

To the left of the answer you chose is a point value — 1, 2 or 3 points. Add up the points from your answers to determine your total score.

10 to 19 points. It's time to put getting into shape on your to-do list. Look for ways to get in 30 minutes or more of physical activity most days, even if it's just 10 minutes at a time.

20 to 25 points. You're on the right track, but your activity level could use a little boost. Look for ways to add more activity to your day or increase the intensity of your activities.

26 to 30 points. Way to go! You're well on your way to maintaining overall fitness. Keep up the good work.

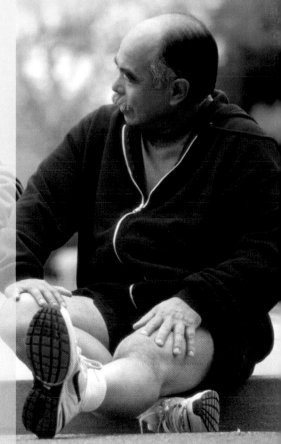

Living a more active life

Physical activity occurs from the moment you slip out of bed in the morning until you crawl back into bed at night. At its most basic level, physical activity simply means moving — every motion of your body burns calories.

Exercise is a more structured approach to physical activity intended to increase fitness.

Both are important. Studies indicate that daily physical activity can provide similar health benefits to structured exercise.

Adding activity to your day

Take advantage of any chance you have to be physically active. Here are a few ideas to help get you started. You can likely think of many other ways to make your day more active.

At home
- Exercise while watching television.
- Wash your car instead of going to the car wash.
- Use a push lawn mower instead of a riding one.
- Rake leaves and spend time in the garden.
- Use hand tools instead of power ones.
- Organize your closets or the garage.

At work
- Park at the far end of the parking lot and walk inside.
- Take the stairs and not the elevator, at least a few floors.
- Get up and visit with your co-workers instead of e-mailing them.
- Walk during your lunch hour.
- Periodically take an activity break. Get up, stretch your legs and move.

When out and about
- Park a little farther from your destination and walk.
- Bike or walk to the store.
- Avoid drive-throughs. Park the car and walk inside.
- Shop. You don't have to buy anything. Just walk the aisles and look at items.
- When golfing, walk the course instead of using a motorized cart.

When with your family
- Take a family walk after enjoying a meal.
- Participate in your kids' activities at the playground or park.
- Plan a family activity at least three times a week. This could be basketball in the driveway or a bike ride.
- Plan vacations that involve physical activities such as hiking, swimming, canoeing or skiing.

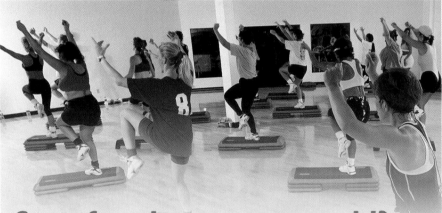

Cure for the common cold?

Researchers at the University of South Carolina in Columbia investigated the relationship between different levels of physical activity and the risk of getting a cold (upper respiratory infection). The study included more than 500 healthy adults between the ages of 20 and 70.

The results found that participants who enjoyed a moderate amount of physical activity experienced 20 percent to 30 percent fewer colds than did individuals whose daily activities were limited and low in intensity.

One possible explanation is that moderate physical activity causes immune system cells to circulate more quickly, enhancing their ability to destroy viruses and bacteria.

Tired of always battling a cold? Get more physical activity each day and see what happens.

Aerobic exercise

One of the simplest and safest forms of exercise — and a great place to start if you're new to exercise — is aerobic activity.

Aerobic means with oxygen, as opposed to *anaerobic*, which means without oxygen. Aerobic activities, such as low to moderately intense walking or swimming, increase your breathing and heart rate as you continuously move your muscles at a regular pace.

Exercises carried out at an intense level placing heavy demands on your muscles and causing them to fatigue quickly are anaerobic. This includes fast running or intense weightlifting.

Both aerobic and anaerobic exercise play a role in achieving fitness. However, the greatest health benefits generally come from aerobic activities.

Beyond the basics

Tired of the same types of exercise? Check out these popular exercises and see what they have to offer:

- Pilates (see page 96)

- Tai chi (see page 100)

- Yoga (see page 101)

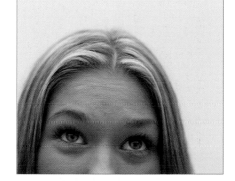

12-week walking program

Walking is an excellent exercise. It's simple, inexpensive, versatile and requires no equipment other than a good pair of walking shoes. If you're new to exercise, try this sample program, in which you slowly progress in the frequency and duration of your walking workout.

Week	Time (minutes)	Days a week	Total hours a week
1	20*	3	1
2	20	3	1
3-4	25	3	1.25
5-6	30	3-4	1.5-2
7-8	35	4-5**	2.5-3
9-10	40	4-5	3-3.5
11-12	40	5-6	3.5-4

*Older adults and people whose fitness is very limited may start out with just five to 10 minutes.

**If the days on which you can exercise are limited, you can continue to walk three or four days a week, instead of increasing the number of days, but gradually extend each walk to 45 or 60 minutes. On the other hand, if you have relatively little time on most days, you may benefit from more frequent but shorter sessions.

This program can be adapted to many ability levels. A beginner might get a sufficient workout from a 10-minute walk around the neighborhood, and a more experienced walker can focus on increasing his or her speed, stride lengths or route, to make the workout more intense. Walking in a hilly area, for instance, may be a good choice for someone looking to boost endurance and build additional muscle tone in his or her legs. Note that walking with hand or ankle weights isn't recommended because adding these weights increases the stress and strain on your body.

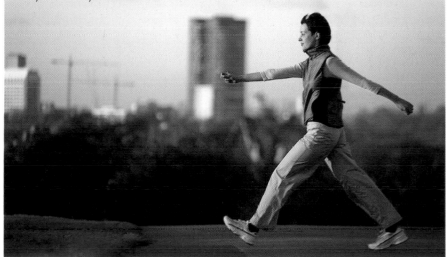

Eat for your health

If you're thinking that a healthy diet means eating bland and boring food, think again.

It's true. You can eat your way to better health. What you put in your mouth every day has a direct effect on how you feel and how your body functions. A healthy diet — one that emphasizes vegetables, fruits and whole grains — may lower your risk of developing many diseases.

If you're thinking that a healthy diet means eating bland and boring foods, think again. It means enjoying great nutrition as well as great taste.

Eating better doesn't need to be complicated. The goal is to eat foods that not only taste good, but are good for you.

Vegetables and fruits

It's hardly news that vegetables and fruits are good for you. The real news is why. Every day more is being learned about how fresh produce supplies the body with a variety of substances to ward off illness.

People who typically eat generous helpings of vegetables and fruits run a lower risk of developing the leading killers of American adults: cardiovascular disease, high blood pressure, cancer and diabetes.

You're not a vegetable and fruit fan? You can be. You just have to know which ones to eat and how to prepare them. For example, instead of the familiar apples and oranges, try kiwi, Bing cherries or mangoes. To add more zest to your vegetables, sprinkle them with herbs.

Remember, much of what you eat is conditioned — that is, over time you've learned to like it. In the same respect, you can learn to enjoy new foods.

Carbohydrates

When it comes to carbohydrates, the key word to remember is *whole*, as in whole grains. The less refined a carbohydrate food is, the better it is for you. Whole grains abound with vitamins, minerals and other important nutrients.

This is why you want to choose whole-grain breads, pastas and cereals whenever you can, and select brown rice instead of white rice.

Contrary to what you may have heard or read, carbohydrates don't make you fat, excess calories do.

Protein and dairy

Despite what you may have learned as a child, it's not necessary to eat meat every day. Although rich in protein, many cuts of meat are high in saturated fat and cholesterol. When you do eat meat, try to eat only lean cuts.

A variety of other foods, including low-fat dairy products, seafood and legumes — dried beans, lentils and peas — furnish protein, too. Try to substitute these foods for meat on a regular basis.

These foods also provide other benefits. Low-fat dairy products are rich in calcium and vitamin D, and seafood supplies omega-3 fatty acids, which help protect against cardiovascular disease.

Fats

Not all fats are bad for you. Nuts, for instance, contain a type of oil that helps keep your heart and arteries free from harmful deposits. And people who replace much of the animal fat in their meals with liquid vegetable oils, such as olive or canola oil, can reduce their blood cholesterol level.

But while nuts and products such as vegetable oil may be beneficial, it's best to use them in moderation. That's because they also contain calories.

Sweets

Yes, it's true, the antioxidants in chocolate — especially dark chocolate — may provide some health benefits. But chocolate also contains plenty of added fat and calories.

When it comes to sweets, small is beautiful. You don't have to give up these foods entirely to eat well, but be smart about your selections and portion sizes.

Make sure you're getting enough antioxidants

Have you ever bitten into an apple, left it on the counter, and returned a few hours later to find it had turned brown? Or left your favorite pruning shears in the garden and discovered them later, covered in rust?

What, you might ask, does that have to do with your health? The answer is simple, although the process is complex: The same chemical reaction that caused the apple to discolor and the shears to rust (oxidation) occurs in your body.

The free radical effect

Your body continuously produces energy at the cellular level by building up and breaking down the substances that you eat and drink. Throughout this process, molecules that are missing an electron are created. These are called free radicals.

Because a free radical doesn't possess a full set of electrons, it's highly unstable and it "steals" an electron from any available substance to put itself in balance. When it does this, it alters the chemical structure of the cell from which it steals.

Free radicals help fight disease and break down toxins, but they're often produced in overabundance, resulting in an imbalance called oxidative stress.

Antioxidants to the rescue

To combat the effects of free radicals, your body produces antioxi-dants. Antioxidants readily give up one of their electrons but continue to stay in balance, sparing nearby cells from the damaging effects of free radicals.

At certain times, such as in the case of shock, infection or exposure to certain substances, naturally occurring antioxidants may not be able to neutralize the effects of all of the free radicals, and cellular damage may occur.

This damage is cumulative, and potentially can lead to degenerative diseases of the nervous system and eye, as well as cancer, diabetes and atherosclerosis.

Increasing your antioxidant intake

You can boost the antioxidants in your body and help fight disease by incorporating foods in your diet that are high in antioxidants — such as those that contain vitamins E, C and carotene, as well as the minerals selenium, copper, zinc and manganese.

Increasing antioxidant levels appears to enhance your health, although no direct link has been confirmed between antioxidant properties of certain foods and the prevention of disease.

Foods naturally highest in antioxidants tend to be those that are rich in color — red, purple, blue, orange and yellow. Dark chocolate, teas and several herbs are also packed with antioxidants.

In addition, how you prepare your foods affects antioxidant levels. For example, more of the antioxidants in tomatoes are available when tomatoes are cooked, whereas broccoli provides more antioxidants when it's raw. In many cases, unpeeled fruits are higher in antioxidants than are peeled forms.

How much is enough?

The Centers for Disease Control and Prevention (CDC) recommends that people eat at least five to seven servings a day of fruits and vegetables. In addition, the CDC recommends four to five servings of nuts, seeds or dry beans a week. All of these foods are good sources of antioxidants.

It's important, though, not to overdo it so that you're consuming a highly excessive amount. Excess consumption of antioxidants beyond your body's ability to use them could lead to increased production of free radicals.

In addition, it's probably best to get your antioxidants from food rather than supplements. Studies of beta carotene supplements indicate they don't protect against heart disease or cancer. To the contrary, they may increase disease risk. Two studies found an increased risk of lung cancer among smokers who took beta carotene supplements, and one found an increased risk of prostate cancer among men who took the supplements and drank alcohol.

10 disease-fighting foods

So then, just what foods should you eat to enjoy great health?

Here are our picks. These 10 foods can lay the groundwork for optimal health.

1. Whole grains

Whole grains are low in fat. And thanks to their fiber content, you eat less because you feel more satisfied. Eating whole grains can help lower your risk of cardiovascular disease, type 2 diabetes and some cancers.

Don't be fooled by the words *wheat bread* or *wheat flour*. Look for the word *whole*. Choose bread or cereal that has whole wheat, whole-wheat flour or another whole grain as the first ingredient on the label.

Look for breads with at least 3 grams of fiber in a serving, or cereals with at least 5 grams of fiber per serving — and preferably 8 or more.

2. Fish

Dietitians recommend that you aim for two servings of fish a week. Broiled, baked or grilled fish are better than fried.

If possible, go for fish such as salmon, tuna, trout, herring and sardines. They're rich in omega-3 fatty acids, which protect against heart disease by improving high-density lipoprotein (HDL or "good") cholesterol and lowering triglycerides. Omega-3s also help lower blood pressure and may reduce the risk of an irregular heartbeat.

However, it's important to pay attention to warnings regarding consumption levels of fish that may be affected by water contaminants, such as mercury and other toxins.

See page 81 for information on fish oil supplements.

3. Walnuts and almonds

Nuts are high in calories but they're also nutrient dense. Almonds are loaded with calcium, iron, natural vitamin E and riboflavin. Walnuts are a good source of phosphorus, zinc, copper, iron, potassium and vitamin E, and are low in saturated fat.

Nuts are naturally cholesterol-free. Studies suggest that they may even help reduce low-density lipoprotein (LDL or "bad") cholesterol and reduce your risk of a heart attack and coronary artery disease.

Eat nuts in moderation. The serving size for nuts is 1 ounce. This equals about 14 walnut halves or about 22 almonds. One serving can take the place of the protein found in 1 ounce of meat.

4. Legumes

Legumes, which include a variety of dried beans, peas and lentils, are high in protein and make an excellent substitute for animal sources of protein.

Legumes have no cholesterol and very little fat. Unlike meat, legumes actually help reduce low-density lipoprotein (LDL or "bad") cholesterol, and the minerals they contain may help control blood pressure.

Add legumes to chili, soups and casseroles in place of meat.

5. Soy

Claims that soy may reduce your cholesterol level and thereby lower your risk of cardiovascular disease are being re-examined after subsequent research found only minimal beneficial effects.

However, soy-based foods are still good for you because they contain less saturated fat than does meat, and they also provide fiber and protein.

It's best to eat soy in moderation, especially if you're at risk of or have had breast cancer. Soy contains phytochemicals that may produce weak estrogen activity. Studies are inconclusive as to whether soy may increase or decrease breast cancer risk.

6. Fat-free dairy products

Fortified skim milk is one of the best ways of getting needed calcium and vitamin D to help prevent osteoporosis.

There's also evidence that calcium can contribute to preventing high blood pressure, stroke, colon cancer and obesity. In addition, milk provides protein, minerals and B vitamins.

Fat-free cottage cheese, fat-free yogurt and fat-free cheeses have similar benefits.

7. Berries

Berries are rich in antioxidants and substances called flavonoids, which may help lower cancer and cardiovascular disease risk.

Blueberries are especially high in antioxidants, but blackberries, raspberries and strawberries aren't far behind.

If you're watching your weight, eat dried fruits sparingly because they're a concentrated source of calories.

8. Broccoli and cauliflower

Both broccoli and cauliflower are high in vitamin C. Broccoli also contains a good amount of vitamin A. These and other cruciferous vegetables — foods such as cabbage, brussels sprouts, bok choy and kale — have naturally occurring phytochemicals that may help reduce the risk of colorectal cancer as well as other cancers. Broccoli and cauliflower also contain fiber, have no cholesterol, and are naturally low in fat and calories.

9. Tomatoes

Tomatoes contain a number of nutrients, including vitamins C and B complex, as well as iron and potassium. They also contain the antioxidant lycopene. Studies indicate that lycopene may lower the risk of heart attack, prostate cancer and possibly other types of cancer.

10. Green tea

Green tea is a major source of phytochemicals known as flavonoids, which may help lower the risk of some diseases.

It's particularly rich in a flavonoid called epigallocatechin gallate, which may inhibit the enzyme activity necessary for some forms of cancer growth.

Although green tea hasn't been shown in laboratory studies to prevent cancer or cardiovascular disease, some evidence suggests it may be of benefit.

Adding color to your meals

Red watermelon, purple grapes and orange sweet potatoes — all are examples of nature's wild color scheme. These bright fruits and vegetables are good for you, too. Different color classes of fruits and vegetables contain varying amounts of plant chemicals (phytochemicals) and other nutrients, offering many health benefits. Try to include these foods in your diet as much as possible.

Color family	Examples	Possible health benefits
Whites, tans, browns include the phytochemical allicin	Garlic, onions, scallions, leeks, bananas, pears, cauliflower	Lowers cholesterol and blood pressure; increases ability to fight infections
Blues, purples include the phytochemicals anthocyanin and phenolics	Blackberries, blueberries, purple grapes, raisins, eggplant, plums	Reduces risk of cancer and heart disease
Deep oranges, bright yellows include the nutrients bioflavonoid and carotenoid	Sweet potatoes, pumpkin, carrots, citrus fruits such as oranges, tangerines, grapefruit	Reduces risk of cancer, heart disease; maintains eyesight; strengthens immune system
Reds include the phytochemicals anthocyanin and lycopene	Tomatoes, watermelon, papaya, pink grapefruit, cherries, red apples, cranberries, red peppers	Reduces risk of heart disease and some cancers
Greens include the phytochemicals lutein and indole	Spinach, romaine lettuce, kale, collards, green peas, kiwi, broccoli, avocado	Protects against vision loss and cancer

Getting in a healthy groove

With everything that you have to do each day, making sure that you and your family eat healthy meals may seem like a difficult or time-consuming task.

When it comes to cooking, many people claim that they don't have the time. That's because healthy eating is often associated with complicated recipes, time-laden meal preparation and hours spent at the grocery store. However, you can prepare a healthy meal as quickly as you can an unhealthy one.

Here are some tips to help you eat well without a lot of fuss and hassle.

Plan by the week

It's more efficient to plan your meals for an entire week, especially if you shop for groceries on a weekly basis. This way, you'll know that you have all of the right ingredients on hand when it's time to prepare breakfast, lunch or dinner.

Look for shortcuts

Another way to help simplify meal preparation and save time is to purchase pre-cut vegetables and fruits, precooked meats and packaged salads.

Frozen or canned vegetables may also come in handy for some dishes. Rinse the canned vegetables to help remove the sodium used in processing.

Shop from a list

Following a list helps keep you from impulse buying. Avoid shopping when you're hungry — you'll be tempted to grab anything that looks vaguely appetizing.

Read nutrition labels

When shopping, compare the nutrition labels of similar items to see if one is healthier than the others. You many find that one has less fat, fewer calories or more fiber.

Adapt to the seasons

Whenever you can, look for recently harvested produce — asparagus, peas and cherries in the spring; peaches, sweet corn and tomatoes in midsummer; and apples, pears and squash in the fall.

In the spring, summer and early fall months, you can find farmers markets in many areas. These markets offer local produce, which tends to be the freshest around.

Be adventurous

Discovering new foods and flavors is part of the joy of cooking and eating, so don't be afraid to explore unfamiliar cuisines. Keep in mind that the broadest range of health benefits comes from meals that feature a wide variety of foods.

Be flexible

Remember that every food you eat doesn't have to be an excellent source of nutrients. Nor is it out of the question to eat high-fat, high-calorie foods on occasion. The main thing is that you choose foods that promote good health more often than you choose those that don't.

Beyond the basics

It may seem easier to reach for a nutritional supplement than eat a healthy diet. However, supplements don't provide many of the benefits of whole foods. Fruits and vegetables, for example, contain naturally occurring food substances called phytochemicals, which may help protect you against cancer, heart disease, diabetes and high blood pressure.

If you depend on dietary supplements rather than eating a variety of whole foods, you miss the benefits of these substances. The best use of supplements is to "supplement" a good diet — not replace it.

For more information on what supplements might be appropriate for you, see Chapter 3.

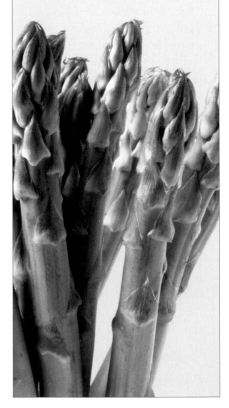

Your weight and your health

Your diet and your weight generally go hand in hand. A healthy diet can help you maintain a healthy weight.

The fact is, the more excess weight you carry, the greater your risk of developing certain health conditions. Among these conditions are:

- **High blood pressure.** Obese individuals are twice as likely to develop high blood pressure (hypertension) as are individuals who maintain a healthy weight.

- **Abnormal blood fats.** Being overweight is associated with low levels of high-density lipoprotein (HDL or "good") cholesterol and high levels of triglycerides (another type of blood fat) in your bloodstream.

- **Type 2 diabetes.** More than 80 percent of adults with type 2 diabetes are over weight or obese.

- **Cardiovascular disease.** A weight gain of just 10 to 20 pounds can increase your risk of heart and blood vessel problems by 25 percent. A gain of 45 pounds or more increases the risk by more than 250 percent.

- **Other complications.** If you're overweight, your health is at increased risk of other conditions, including osteoarthritis, gallstones and sleep apnea. Many types of cancer also are associated with being overweight.

The right approach

If you really want to lose weight and keep the weight off, the best approach is to focus on healthy lifestyle changes and to follow an eating plan that's enjoyable, yet healthy and low in calories.

This approach will result in weight loss that you can live with — that is, that you can maintain over a long period of time. What you don't want is to gain the weight back.

True, achieving a healthy weight takes work — or more correctly, planning — but the rewards are great. Your efforts will result in a sustainable, enjoyable lifestyle that can improve your health and well-being. You'll feel better immediately and at the same time reduce your health risks.

Slow and steady wins the race

That there are so many diet plans to choose from these days attests to the fact that few of them work for most people or are effective for a long period of time. The term *diet* often implies something that's restrictive and negative and, therefore, temporary. Many diets will help people lose weight over a short period of time, but usually the weight is regained. People often find diets hard to sustain because they get tired of avoiding certain foods, loading up on others or feeling deprived and hungry.

Weight loss is best — and most likely to be retained — when it's gradual and it results from a change in lifestyle habits. Think in terms of losing no more than 1 to 2 pounds a week. That's a goal that's realistic and achievable. A loss of just 5 percent to 10 percent of your body weight — no matter what you weigh — brings important health benefits and improves the quality of your life.

Here's a practical perspective on weight loss: 3,500 calories equals about 1 pound of body fat. To lose 1 pound in a week, you need to burn 3,500 calories more than you consume. That calculates to about 500 fewer calories a day. How do you do this? Eat fewer high-calorie foods, get more physical activity or, better yet, do both.

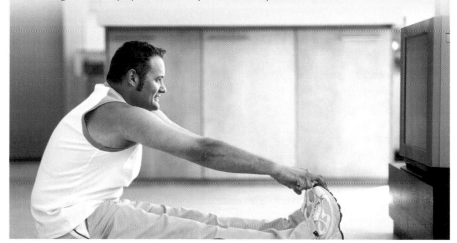

Find meaning in your life

Enjoying life is about taking part in activities and relationships that are meaningful to you — that motivate you to get up every morning.

Good health, remember, is more than your physical health, it also includes your mental health. Increasing evidence suggests that how you view life and the satisfaction you get from life have a major influence on your health.

If you're happy in what you're doing and you feel that your life has meaning and purpose, you're more likely to enjoy a healthy life. Without a sense of mission — a passion for something or someone — some people become vulnerable to depression or other illnesses.

Relationships

Strong social ties are one component of a purposeful life. Healthy relationships with family and friends appear to boost your physical health in a number of ways:

- **Bolster immunity.** Stress can suppress immunity. To the contrary, love and friendship reduce stress and strengthen immunity.
- **Improve mental health.** Having people to talk with provides a psychological buffer against stress, anxiety and depression.
- **Improve recovery.** Studies suggest that individuals who

Increasing evidence suggests that how you view life and the satisfaction that you get from life have a major influence on your health.

have a strong support system are likely to recover faster from a major health event than those who don't.

- **Extend life.** More than a dozen studies link social support with a lower risk of early death.

Activities

Another component of a purposeful life is spending your days doing what you enjoy.

A feeling of satisfaction comes in many different forms. For some individuals, their job provides meaning and enjoyment. Others find satisfaction in raising their children or caring for family members. For still others, real meaning in life may come from a hobby or civic duty.

Remember, satisfaction doesn't have to come in big packages. Something as simple as having coffee with friends may be what you look forward to and what gives you pleasure.

Spiritual ties

Similar to the benefits that come from strong relationships and meaningful activities, spiritual well-being is integral to health and happiness.

People often use the term *spirituality* interchangeably with

religion. However, the terms aren't necessarily synonymous. Whereas religion refers to a system of beliefs and practices held by a group of believers, spirituality is more individualistic and self-determined.

Praying is one means of expressing your spirituality. Other activities people find to be spiritually soothing include spending time in nature or enjoying the pleasures of music, art or writing.

Spiritual beliefs and practices — whatever form they may take — help you connect to something greater than yourself. When you believe in some form of higher power, you strengthen your ability to cope with whatever life hands you.

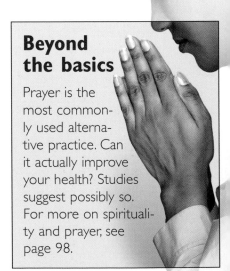

Beyond the basics

Prayer is the most commonly used alternative practice. Can it actually improve your health? Studies suggest possibly so. For more on spirituality and prayer, see page 98.

A healthy marriage: Why love is good for you

One example of how relationships affect health is marriage. The relationship between health and marriage has been studied for decades. Statistics show that people who are happily married live longer than do their single counterparts. They have lower rates of heart failure, cancer and other diseases and they develop tighter networks of emotional support.

According to one study, married women are 20 percent less likely than are single women to die of a variety of causes, including heart disease, suicide and cirrhosis of the liver. Married men enjoy an even greater benefit — they're two to three times less likely to die of such causes than are single men.

The upsides of a healthy marriage — one that includes a strong commitment and open lines of communication — span both mental and emotional well-being.

While the benefits of marriage may be clear, the reason married couples live healthier lives is more elusive. The prevailing explanation has to do with less stress.

Marriage and stress

The detrimental effect of stress on an individual's health is well-known. Cardiovascular, hormonal and immune pathways are important to a person's well-being, and stress can negatively affect these systems.

Experts reason that married couples enjoy better health partly because they're better equipped as a team to handle and defray stress than are their single counterparts.

Aspects of a healthy marriage thought to ease stress include:

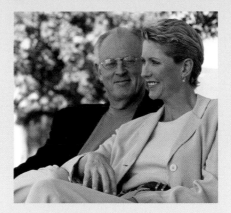

More money

By pooling their incomes, married couples amass greater wealth over a lifetime than do single people. Further, there are economies of cohabitation. A married couple can live more cheaply than can a single person by sharing housing costs, utilities, groceries and insurance.

Expanded support network

A healthy marriage brings together two teams of friends and family, thereby multiplying the support network upon which a couple can rely to tackle life's ups and downs. This can translate into not only physical but mental health benefits.

Improved behaviors

People make different choices and adopt different behaviors once they're married. Healthy activities generally increase, and risky behaviors typically decrease, partly due to a sense of responsibility to a spouse and children.

A Centers for Disease Control and Prevention (CDC) study found that married adults are about half as likely to be smokers as are single, divorced or separated adults. They're also less likely to be heavy drinkers or engage in risky sexual behavior.

The lone exception is weight control. Studies show that married adults, particularly men, weigh more and have higher rates of obesity than do single adults. People who have never been married are the least likely to be overweight.

A committed relationship

Unmarried couples in a committed relationship also appear to enjoy similar health gains. However, the CDC study indicates that unmarried couples generally don't reap as high a level of health benefits as do married couples.

Why the difference? Researchers don't know for certain. One theory is that unmarried couples may have a weaker network of social support than do married couples. However, other factors may also be involved.

An unhealthy marriage

Just as a healthy marriage provides a host of benefits, an unhealthy one can have negative health consequences in that it can be an enormous source of stress.

A study of newlywed couples conducted at The Ohio State University found that hostile and negative behavior was associated with a decline in immune system response. This can spur a number of health consequences, such as slower wound healing and greater susceptibility to infectious disease.

Take time to rest and relax

Rest and relaxation are basic necessities. They're as fundamental to your health as physical activity and a nutritious diet.

If you're like many people, though, you don't get enough. And your body is paying for it.

Not enough rest and too little sleep can make it more difficult for you to concentrate, and you may become impatient with others, less interactive in your relationships and less productive at work.

Benefits of rest and relaxation

When it comes to your health, it's important to make sleep and relaxation a priority. Each day you may feel the need to complete a long list of tasks, and then with whatever time is leftover, sleep or relax.

Try this: Reverse the order. Set aside adequate time for sleep and relaxation and then see how many of the tasks on your list you can get done in the time you have remaining. You may be surprised.

There are many reasons why relaxation and a good night's sleep are important to your health. They:

- Slow your heart rate, meaning less work for your heart
- Reduce your blood pressure
- Increase blood flow to your major muscles
- Slow your breathing rate

- Lessen muscle tension
- Reduce signs and symptoms of illness, such as headaches, nausea, diarrhea and pain
- Give you more energy
- Improve your concentration

Tips for better sleep

If you have trouble sleeping, simple changes in your daily and bedtime routines may make sleep come easier. Here are a few suggestions:

- **Stick to a sleep schedule.** Go to bed and get up about the same time every day, including weekends.
- **Establish and follow a bedtime ritual.** In the evening, slow the pace of your activities before bedtime.
- **Exercise and stay active.** Physical activity enhances deep and refreshing sleep. But avoid exercising too close to bedtime.
- **Create a comfortable sleep environment.** Keep your bedroom quiet, dark and comfortably cool.
- **Don't eat too close to bedtime.** Having a full stomach increases your chances of experiencing heartburn while lying in bed.
- **Avoid or limit caffeine and alcohol.** Caffeine can prevent you from falling asleep.

Alcohol can cause shallow sleeping and frequent awakenings.
- **Don't 'try' to sleep.** If sleep doesn't come naturally, read a book, listen to music or watch television until you feel drowsy.

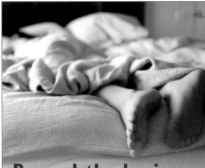

Beyond the basics

In upcoming pages, you'll read about a number of techniques that can help you relax and reduce stress. These include:

- Biofeedback (see page 86)
- Guided imagery (see page 87)
- Massage (see page 117)
- Meditation (see page 90)
- Muscle relaxation (see page 94)
- Music therapy (see page 95)
- Relaxed breathing (see page 97)
- Yoga (see page 101)

To sleep better, check out:
- Melatonin (see page 80)
- Valerian (see page 66)

Address stress

Modern-day life is full of time pressures and demands. In other words, it's stressful. But just because stress may be a regular component of your day, it doesn't have to get the best of you.

Too much stress

Many of the physical reactions that accompany stress can damage your long-term health. Stress can be a factor in a variety of illnesses, from headaches to heart disease. Stress may aggravate an existing health problem, or it may trigger an illness if you're already at risk.

- **Immune system.** The hormone cortisol produced during times of stress can suppress your immune system, increasing your susceptibility to infections, including upper respiratory infections such as cold or flu.

- **Cardiovascular disease.** During acute stress your heart beats more quickly, making you more susceptible to heart-rhythm irregularities and chest pain (angina). If you're a "hot reactor" or a "Type A" personality, acute stress may increase your heart attack risk. Increased blood clotting from persistent stress also can put you at risk of a heart attack or stroke.

- **Other illnesses.** Other relationships between illness and stress are less clear cut, but stress may worsen symptoms of asthma, irritable bowel syndrome, skin disorders, chronic pain, depression or anxiety.

How to stress less

There are many ways to deal with stress. You may find it helpful to talk about your problems, listen to some soothing music or sit in a warm bathtub or hot tub.

You might also experiment with activities intended to help you relax, such as meditation, relaxed breathing, visualization or yoga. These relaxation techniques are discussed in upcoming pages.

Good health will also help you combat stress. Get adequate sleep, keep physically active and eat well.

Good stress

Not all stress is bad. Stress can result from both negative and positive situations. Negative stress occurs when you feel out of control or under constant or intense pressure. Too much negative stress is damaging. Stress brought on by a positive cause — the birth of a child or a new job — provides a feeling of excitement and opportunity. Positive stress helps challenge and motivate us.

Life without any stress would be boring. The key is to experience more good stress than bad.

Signs and symptoms of stress overload

Physical	Thoughts and feelings	Behaviors
Headache	Excessive worrying	Overeating or appetite loss
Chest pain	Anxiety	Increased arguing
Pounding heart	Anger	Angry outbursts
High blood pressure	Irritability	Increased alcohol and drug use
Shortness of breath	Depression	Increased smoking
Muscle aches	Sadness	Withdrawal or isolation
Clenched jaws	Restlessness	Crying spells
Grinding teeth	Mood swings	Neglecting responsibility
Tight, dry throat	Feeling insecure	Decreased productivity
Indigestion	Difficulty concentrating	Job dissatisfaction
Diarrhea or constipation	Confusion	Poor job performance
Stomach cramping	Forgetfulness	Increased use of sick time
Increased perspiration	Resentment	Burnout
Fatigue	Tendency to blame	Impatience
Insomnia	Negativity	Change in sleep patterns
Weight gain or loss	Guilt	Changes in relationships
Skin problems	Apathy	Nervous twitch or habit
Impaired sexual function	Feeling worthless	Decreased interest in sex

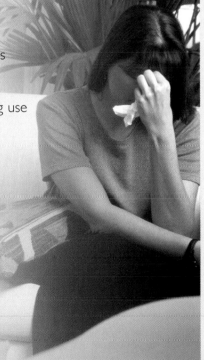

Part 2

Guide to Complementary & Alternative Therapies

Understanding the benefits and risks of popular treatments

Complementary and alternative medicine includes a diverse group of products, practices and therapies intended to treat and prevent illness.

As these treatments increasingly undergo scientific study, some are gradually incorporated into mainstream medicine, while others fall out of favor because they're considered ineffective or unsafe. For a number of complementary and alternative treatments, the jury is still out — either research results have been inconclusive or not enough research has been done to determine the effectiveness or safety of the therapy.

In Part 2, we take a look at various forms of alternative and complementary medicine and provide you with the latest information on what's known about the treatments — their benefits and their risks. We also offer information on how to incorporate specific treatments into your daily life.

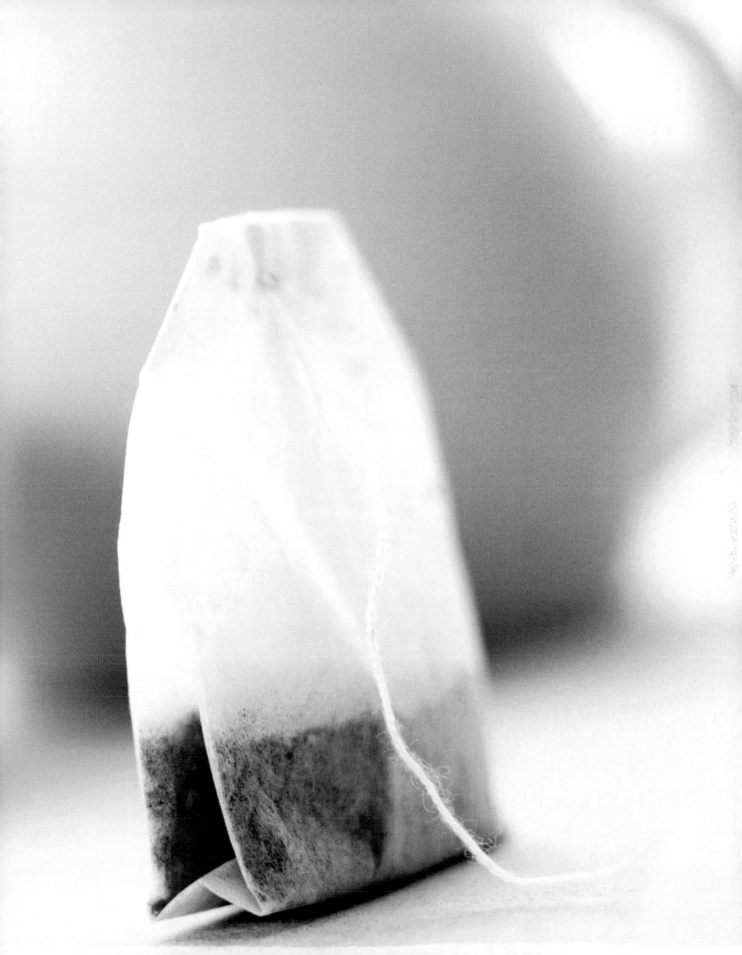

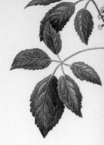

Our top 10

As we begin the section on complementary and alternative therapies, here's a brief rundown of what we consider to be the 10 best therapies at this point in time.

Research into complementary and alternative medicine is rapidly evolving. New studies are coming forward on an increasingly frequent basis and, many times, new studies conflict with older studies. To complicate matters even more, different forms can have different effects. This makes it difficult to state with authority which therapies are truly "the best." However, we've listed what we consider to be the top 10.

Therapy	What it's most commonly used for
Acupuncture	Nausea, fibromyalgia, and some forms of dental, post-surgical and chronic pain (see page 106)
Guided imagery	Headache and some forms of pain (see page 87)
Hypnosis	Anxiety, pain and tension headache (see page 89)
Massage	Anxiety, back pain and fibromyalgia (see page 117)
Meditation	Anxiety, stress, fibromyalgia and high blood pressure (see page 90)
Music therapy	Relaxation, stress and depression (see page 95)
Spinal manipulation	Low back pain (see page 122)
Spirituality	Medical illness and chronic disease (see page 98)
Tai chi	Balance and strength and cardiovascular disease (see page 100)
Yoga	Anxiety, stress, depression, heart disease, and high blood pressure (see page 101)

Leading contenders

You'll notice that in our top 10 list we didn't include any dietary supplements. That's not because supplements don't provide benefits — many of them do, and we're learning more about their potential uses every day. The trouble is, most dietary supplements haven't gone through rigorous study to fully determine their effectiveness and their safety. And because supplements carry risk of harm — as does any medication — it's difficult to place these products in a top 10 list until more is known about them.

We do believe, however, that there are a number of products that hold promise and we expect to hear more about them in coming years.

Supplement	What it's most commonly taken for
Black cohosh	Hot flashes (see page 45)
Chondroitin	Arthritis (see page 78)
Garlic	High cholesterol (see page 52)
Ginkgo	Dementia and claudication (see page 53)
Ginseng	Improved quality of life (see page 54)
Glucosamine	Arthritis (see page 78)
St. John's wort	Mild depression (see page 65)
SAM-e	Arthritis and depression (see page 82)
Saw palmetto	Benign prostatic hyperplasia (see page 63)
Valerian	Sleep difficulties and anxiety (see page 66)

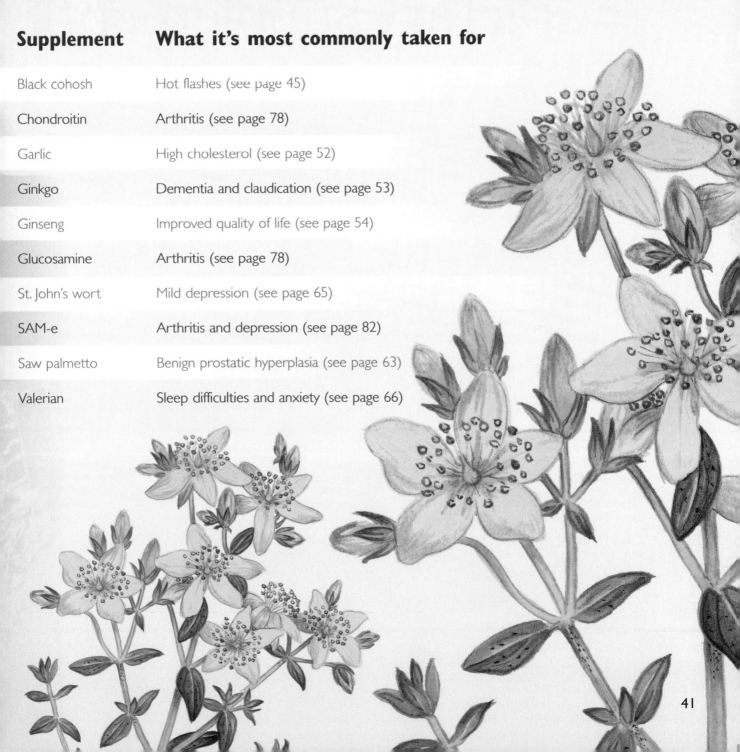

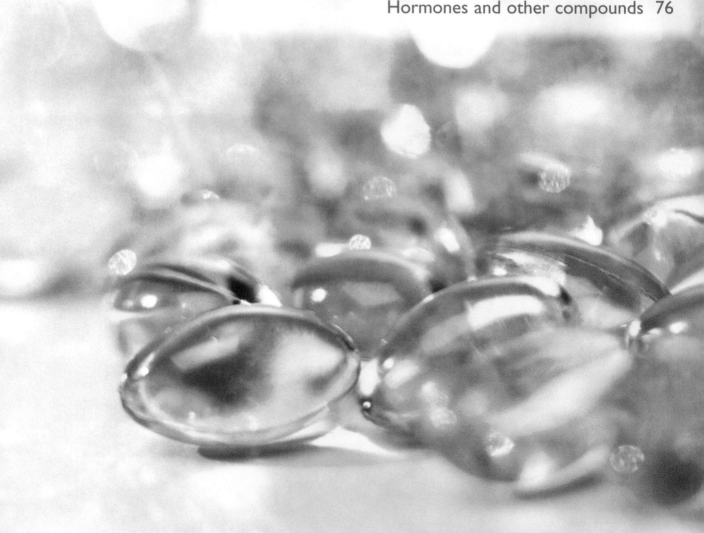

Chapter 3
Herbs and Other Dietary Supplements

A visit with Dr. Mark Lee

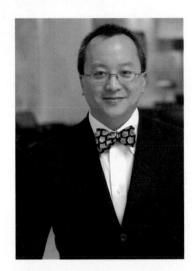

Mark Lee, M.D.
General Internal Medicine

There's growing evidence that certain supplements — when used in conjunction with modern medicine — can help you achieve and maintain good health. Supplements can be part of your overall wellness plan, provided you use them wisely. "

The most common alternative therapy in use today is dietary supplements, which include herbs, vitamins and minerals. Since 1994, when the U.S. Congress passed the Dietary Supplement Health and Education Act, there's been a tremendous explosion of growth in the dietary supplement industry, with sales exceeding $20 billion annually, according to some estimates.

Most dietary supplements are derived from plants or herbs, though minerals, vitamins and even some hormones, such as DHEA and melatonin, are included in the category. People often take supplements because they believe that taking them is good for the prevention and treatment of many diseases, including arthritis, osteoporosis, infections and immune-related conditions. Supplements — especially herbal products — are also popular because of the perception that they're natural and, therefore, "good for you." But natural doesn't always translate into being safe. Any product that's strong enough to provide a potential benefit to the body can also be strong enough to cause harm. Tobacco, for example, is a "natural" product, and it's clearly not safe. Some natural products, such as nightshade or hemlock, can be extremely toxic when ingested and can even cause death.

Vitamins have generally proved to be safe. However, marketing campaigns and the antioxidant craze of the past decade have spurred the concept that "if a little is good for you, then a lot must be great." Megadose vitamin therapies are publicized as effective strategies to cure colds and infections, prevent Alzheimer's disease, and even prevent or cure cancer. Unfortunately, there's little scientific evidence to support these claims and their side effects have resulted in more of a problem rather than a panacea.

Despite these concerns, there's growing evidence that certain supplements — when used in conjunction with modern medicine — can help you achieve and maintain good health. Supplements can be part of your overall wellness plan, provided you use them wisely. When reading supplement labels, ask yourself these questions: Does the product promise rapid improvement in health or performance? Does it seem too good to be true? Does the manufacturer use the results of a single study or series of anecdotes to support its use?

And remember, supplements are just that — supplemental. They can't replace a nutritious diet. To achieve and maintain good health, you need to build your "health pyramid" — don't smoke, eat nutritious foods, exercise every day, rest up and make sure to have meaning in your life. Once you've created and maintained this foundation, adding specific supplements may provide the added edge you're looking for.

Promise and peril

Dietary supplements may be popular, but are they right for you? That depends on the product, your current health and your medical history.

Dietary supplements contain ingredients that affect how your body functions, just as nonprescription and prescription medications do. Some supplements may be beneficial, but in other instances herbal supplements may be risky. Their labels are often vague, and the supplement may pose more unwanted side effects than benefits.

If you're considering a dietary supplement, educate yourself about the product you intend to use before purchasing it, and talk to your doctor about the supplement you're considering taking.

It's wise to avoid dietary supplements if:

- **You're pregnant or breast-feeding.** As a general rule, don't take any medications when you're pregnant or breast-feeding unless your doctor approves. Medications that may be safe for you as an adult may be harmful to your fetus or your breast-feeding infant.
- **You're having surgery.** Many herbal supplements can affect the success of surgery. Some may decrease the effectiveness of anesthetics or cause dangerous complications such as bleeding or high blood pressure. Tell your doctor about any herbs you're taking or considering taking as soon as you know you need surgery.

- **You're younger than 18 or older than 65.** Older adults may metabolize medications differently. And few herbal supplements have been tested on children or have established safe doses for children. While it's recommended that all individuals consult with a doctor before taking dietary supplements, it's especially important that you do so if:
- **You're taking prescription or nonprescription medications.** Some herbs can cause serious side effects when mixed with prescription or nonprescription drugs, such as aspirin. Talk to your doctor about possible drug interactions.

More information on supplement safety can be found in Chapter 9.

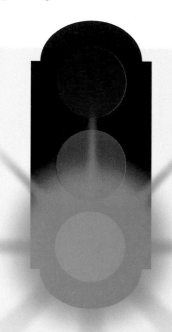

What a green light means

In upcoming pages, you'll find herbs and other supplements that have been given a green light. Remember that a green light doesn't mean it's OK to take the product for any condition or in any amount. Oftentimes, a product is given a green light because studies have found it beneficial for just one or two conditions. There may be other conditions for which it isn't effective. Always take the product according to directions. Don't take more than is recommended, and always discuss your use of supplements with your doctor. You'll note that we usually advise not to take the product for more than six months. This is because — with some exceptions — most products haven't been studied for longer than six months to determine their long-term effects.

Herbs and other botanicals

Black cohosh

Black cohosh (*Actaea racemosa*), formerly known as *Cimicifuga racemosa*, is a member of the buttercup family. It's also called black snakeroot and bugbane.

Because it has effects similar to the female hormone estrogen, black cohosh is used to relieve premenstrual pain and symptoms of menopause. In the past, it was also used to treat rheumatic joint pain.

Black cohosh is generally well tolerated, but it can cause stomach discomfort. The safety and efficacy of long-term treatment is still unknown.

Our take
We give black cohosh a green light because it may improve menopausal symptoms, especially hot flashes, if used in recommended doses. Don't take it for longer than six months. For other conditions, there's less evidence it may be beneficial, so be cautious.

What the research says
Several controlled trials report that black cohosh improves menopausal symptoms such as hot flashes, headache and mood disorders. There are also indications it may relieve heart palpitations and sleep disturbances. However, many of these studies were small, weakly designed and didn't extend beyond six months. There are no quality studies to indicate it relieves arthritis or other forms of joint pain.

Butterbur

Butterbur (*Petasites hybridus*) is a shrub found along marshy meadows and riversides. Its name comes from its large, supple leaves that were used to wrap butter before the days of refrigeration.

There's evidence that butterbur may help prevent migraines and treat hay fever (allergic rhinitis). This may be due to its anti-inflammatory properties and its ability to relax blood vessel walls.

People who are allergic to ragweed, marigolds and daisies need to be especially cautious if taking this supplement.

Our take
Butterbur gets a green light because the herb appears to be relatively safe if taken for a short period to help prevent migraines or to treat symptoms of hay fever. However, don't take butterbur for either of these conditions without first consulting with your doctor, to prevent possible drug interactions.

What the research says
Some studies indicate participants who took butterbur were able to significantly decrease the number of migraine attacks. Other studies suggest that butterbur may alleviate the stuffiness and nasal congestion of hay fever. However, due to the small sample sizes and short durations of these studies, the results can only be considered preliminary. Additional research is needed.

Cat's claw

Cat's claw (*Uncaria tomentosa*) is a woody vine from the tropical rainforests of Central and South America. Its name comes from hooked thorns that run along the vine's surface.

The plant was highly prized among various indigenous groups in the Americas for its medicinal properties. Today, it's used to boost the immune system and to treat inflammatory conditions as well as cancer.

Cat's claw may lower your blood pressure, so if you're taking antihypertensive drugs, talk to your doctor before taking the supplement.

Our take

Preliminary studies suggest a possible role for cat's claw in treating ailments such as rheumatoid arthritis and osteoarthritis; however the evidence still isn't strong enough to recommend it. There's less evidence it can help boost the immune system. The full potential of its medicinal qualities awaits further study.

What the research says

Studies indicate modest benefits for easing joint pain from rheumatoid arthritis, as well as osteoarthritic knee pain during physical activity (but not during rest). However, these studies were limited in size and additional research is necessary before the use of cat's claw can be recommended for either condition.

As for its role as an immune system booster, a few small studies have produced conflicting results.

Cayenne

Originating in the Americas, the hot, fiery cayenne pepper (*Capsicum annuum*) is known in kitchens around the world as red pepper or chili pepper.

The bright red fruit of the plant contains an ingredient called capsaicin, which has been found to deplete nerve cells of a chemical that helps transmit pain messages.

Applied as a cream, cayenne is used to relieve joint and muscle pain. It's also taken in tablet form to help relieve gastrointestinal problems.

Make sure to keep the cream away from your eyes, nose and mouth. Wash your hands thoroughly after application.

Our take

We give cayenne a green light because it can be an effective topical pain reliever for rheumatoid arthritis and osteoarthritis, as well as for nerve damage caused by the complications of diabetes. Follow label directions. For other conditions, be cautious. The evidence still isn't there to support its use.

What the research says

Several studies support the use of topical cayenne for pain relief, especially to joints located close to the skin's surface, such as fingers, knees and elbows.

There have been fewer studies done on cayenne taken in pill form. It may have some therapeutic benefit for gastrointestinal problems, but there are no studies supporting its effectiveness.

Chasteberry

Chasteberry (*Vitex agnus-castus*) is the peppery fruit of a tree that's native to the Mediterranean region. Long thought to inspire chastity, it earned the name "monk's pepper" in the Middle Ages.

Chasteberry is most commonly used to treat hormone-related problems in women.

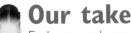

Our take

Early research suggests chasteberry may be an effective treatment for premenstrual syndrome (PMS). While the herb appears relatively safe, its full effects aren't known. Use it with caution.

What the research says

In clinical trials, chasteberry reduced some signs and symptoms of PMS, especially breast pain or tenderness, swelling, constipation and mood changes. It can cause gastrointestinal upset, headache and itching.

Cinnamon

In addition to a kitchen spice, cinnamon is used in traditional medicine. The variety *Cinnamomum cassia* is the one most often used in natural remedies and found to be most effective for lowering blood sugar.

People take cinnamon to help control type 2 diabetes. It's also used for digestive disorders, and appears in lotions, mouthwashes and toothpaste.

Our take

Cinnamon is safe for general use, but it needs more study. The cinnamon sold for cooking and baking generally contains a mixture of different varieties. You don't know how much — if any — *Cinnamomum cassia* you're getting. Don't set aside proven diabetes medications for cinnamon.

What the research says

Several studies have suggested that compounds in cinnamon may make cells more responsive to insulin, which would be of great value to people with type 2 diabetes. However, a recent small study found that cinnamon supplements had little effect on insulin sensitivity among postmenopausal women.

Devil's claw

Devil's claw (*Harpagophytum procumbens*) has been used in the traditional medicine of people of the Kalahari Desert in southern Africa.

Devil's claw is used to relieve pain and inflammation in joints and to treat headache and back pain. The manner in which it works is unknown.

Our take

Devil's claw is used extensively in Europe and appears to be effective as an anti-inflammatory agent for treating osteoarthritis and low back pain. There's no known benefit for rheumatoid arthritis.

What the research says

Studies suggest devil's claw is effective in the short-term treatment of osteoarthritic pain. Separate trials indicate that it may also help alleviate low back pain. Additional study is needed before more definitive recommendations can be made.

Echinacea

You may know echinacea by its common name, the coneflower. It belongs to the same plant family as the sunflower, thistle and black-eyed Susan.

The roots and herbs from three echinacea species are prepared for medicinal use as pills, applications and teas. The most popular is *Echinacea purpurea*, or the purple coneflower.

Echinacea traditionally has been used to treat everything from skin wounds to dizziness to cancer. In the 20th century, it became an extremely popular remedy for colds and flu.

Recent interest in echinacea is due to its purported ability to boost the immune system — in particular, its ability to fight colds and upper respiratory tract infections.

The use of echinacea is popular and growing. In the United States, sales of echinacea may represent about 10 percent of the dietary supplement market.

Because the active ingredient hasn't been identified, there's often a problem with quality control. Some products may contain very small amounts of echinacea, if any at all.

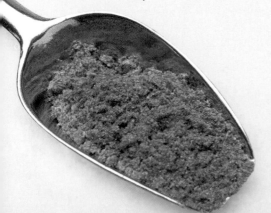

Our take

Unfortunately, there's still no cure for the common cold. Despite all of the claims, latest study results suggest echinacea isn't an effective method for cold prevention or treatment, as once thought. If you have a cold, it won't hurt you to try echinacea for a few days, but there's no guarantee that it will help. Don't use it for more than eight weeks at a time. As for other claims, the research isn't there yet. It's unclear whether echinacea can boost the immune system.

What the research says

Here's what some studies of echinacea have found:

Cancer

There's no clear evidence that echinacea has an effect on any type of cancer in humans.

Immune system booster

Echinacea has been studied alone and in combination with other ingredients for its effect on the immune system — including people receiving chemotherapy for cancer. It's still unclear if there are any significant benefits. Definitive conclusions will require additional studies regarding safety and effectiveness.

Upper respiratory tract infections

A number of uncontrolled studies suggested that adults could reduce the length and severity of a cold by taking echinacea orally at the first sign of symptoms. However, a 2005 clinical trial reported no such benefits. It may be that other echinacea preparations not tested in this study could provide some benefit. Initial research also suggests that echinacea doesn't alleviate cold symptoms in children, as once thought.

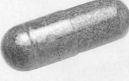

Other

Studies of echinacea as a treatment for genital herpes and low white blood cell counts following X-ray treatment found no apparent benefits.

Ephedra

Ephedra sinica, or ma-huang, is an evergreen shrub native to the Central Asian desert. It contains the alkaloids ephedrine and pseudoephedrine, which stimulate the central nervous system. Ephedra became a popular remedy for colds, asthma and bronchitis, and it's frequently combined with caffeine in medications to promote weight loss.

The sale of dietary supplements containing ephedra was prohibited due to safety concerns. The ban has been appealed on the grounds that risks have not been proved when ephedra is taken at lower doses — that the safety concerns were associated with higher doses or when ephedra is used in combination with caffeine. To date, the ban is still being upheld; however, ephedra products are available on the Internet.

Our take

We don't recommend ephedra for treatment of obesity or any other condition because it can be dangerous. Serious cardiovascular side effects may occur if the herb is taken at higher doses.

What the research says

Ephedra is most commonly taken for weight loss. It also was once a popular treatment for asthma.

Asthma

Ephedra became a popular treatment for childhood asthma in the 1920s because of its ability to relax the bronchial air passages. Since then, better asthma medications have been developed. Ephedra also is considered too risky because it can cause serious side effects, and commercial products may contain variable concentrations of the herb — either too much or too little.

Weight loss

Ephedrine used in combination with caffeine appears to promote weight loss. But studies to date have been small and not of good quality. They also have suffered from high drop-out rates due to side effects. In studies in which ephedrine was taken alone, without caffeine, participants experienced little if any weight loss.

Herbs to watch out for

Some herbs may pose serious health risks. Here is a listing of herbs considered to be dangerous, either because of their potential for serious side effects or because overdoses can be fatal: alpine ragwort, herbs that contain aristolochic acid (such as wild ginger), belladonna, bitter orange, chaparral, coltsfoot, comfrey, ephedra, germander, golden ragwort (life root), goldenseal, kava, licorice root, lobelia, pennyroyal, Scotch broom, skullcap and yohimbe. This list isn't complete — there may be others.

Keep in mind that dangerous herbs may be mixed into products that contain a combination of herbs. That's why it's important to read the label on all products so that you know what you're taking.

For more information on safe use of herbal and other dietary supplements, see Chapter 9.

Herbal weight-loss products: Do they work?

The appeal of quick weight loss with the help of over-the-counter weight-loss pills is often hard to pass up. But are they a safe option for weight loss? And do they do anything but lighten your wallet?

The accompanying chart provides a summary of some popular over-the-counter weight-loss pills and what they will — and won't — do for you.

Dietary supplements and weight-loss aids aren't subject to the same rigorous standards as are prescription drugs or medications sold over-the-counter. Therefore, they can be marketed with limited proof of effectiveness or safety.

Many weight-loss pills contain a cocktail of ingredients — some with more than 20 herbs, botanicals, vitamins, minerals or other add-ons. How these ingredients interact individually and collectively with your body is largely unknown. Using them can be a risky venture.

Keep in mind, there's no magic bullet for losing weight. Even if these products were to help you lose weight initially, you'd have to continue taking them for the weight to stay off, which is neither practical nor safe.

Supplement	The claims	What you need to know
Bitter orange	Decreases appetite	• Touted as an "ephedra substitute" but may cause health problems similar to those of ephedra • Long-term effects unknown
Chitosan	Blocks absorption of dietary fat	• Relatively safe, but unlikely to cause weight loss • Can cause constipation, bloating and other gastrointestinal complaints • Long-term effects unknown
Chromium	Reduces body fat and builds muscle	• Relatively safe, but unlikely to build muscle or cause weight loss • Long-term effects unknown
Conjugated linoleic acid (CLA)	Reduces body fat, decreases appetite and builds muscle	• Might decrease body fat and increase muscle, but it isn't likely to reduce total weight • Can cause diarrhea, indigestion and other gastrointestinal problems
Country mallow (heartleaf)	Decreases appetite and increases the number of calories burned	• Contains ephedrine, which is dangerous • Likely unsafe and should be avoided
Ephedra	Decreases appetite	• Can cause high blood pressure, heart rate irregularities, sleeplessness, seizures, heart attacks, strokes and even death • Banned because of safety concerns
Green tea extract	Increases calorie and fat metabolism and decreases appetite	• Limited evidence to support claim • Can cause vomiting, bloating, indigestion and diarrhea • May contain a large amount of caffeine
Guar gum	Blocks absorption of dietary fat and increases the feeling of fullness, which leads to decreased calorie intake	• Relatively safe, but unlikely to cause weight loss • Can cause diarrhea and other gastrointestinal problems
Hoodia	Decreases appetite	• No conclusive evidence to support claim

Feverfew

Feverfew (*Tanacetum parthenium*) is a member of the daisy family, also known as bachelor's button or midsummer daisy. It has been used for centuries to fight fever, headache and menstrual irregularity.

Generally, the feverfew leaf is prepared as a powder or tablet. The active ingredient, partheolide, seems to make the cerebral blood vessels less reactive to chemicals that may cause headaches.

Our take

If you suffer from migraines and aren't helped by medication, you may want to give feverfew a try to see if you notice any benefits. However, do so only under a doctor's supervision, don't take more than the recommended amount and don't take it for more than six months. Be aware that feverfew may cause an allergic reaction in people sensitive to flowers such as daisies and marigolds.

What the research says

Studies indicate that feverfew, taken at the recommended daily amount, can reduce the frequency of migraine attacks. However, these studies were set up for 24 weeks or less, and the effects of long-term usage remains unknown. Better designed trials with other migraine therapies are necessary.

Evidence that the herb is beneficial in the treatment of rheumatoid arthritis is inconclusive.

Gamma linolenic acid

Gamma linolenic acid (GLA) is an omega-6 fatty acid. It's necessary for good health, but it isn't produced in the body.

The body obtains GLA from the breakdown of certain foods during digestion. GLA supplements are available from seed extracts of black currant, borage and evening primrose.

GLA is converted in the body to compounds with anti-inflammatory properties. It's used to treat a wide range of conditions, including rheumatoid arthritis, inflammation of the skin (dermatitis), nerve damage due to diabetes and ulcerative colitis.

Our take

We give gamma linolenic acid a green light because it appears to help prevent nerve damage (peripheral neuropathy) from diabetes. There really is no better alternative treatment for this condition, and GLA appears to be relatively safe. But make sure to follow label directions.

For treatment of other conditions, such as rheumatoid arthritis, there's not enough evidence that it works.

What the research says

Two good-quality studies indicate that GLA may help prevent nerve damage in people with diabetes. Additional and larger studies are needed to confirm this result.

There's some evidence that GLA may be useful in the treatment of rheumatoid arthritis but, again, more study is needed. Benefits are not apparent for the treatment of dermatitis.

Garlic

Garlic (*Allium sativum*) is a member of the lily family and a close relative of the onion. It's been used for centuries to treat conditions ranging from high blood pressure to tumors to protection from snake venom.

Garlic appears to have many effects on the cardiovascular system. It's most effective when you eat it raw and in large amounts, but it can also be purchased in tablet form.

Don't use garlic if you're taking anti-clotting drugs because garlic can increase risk of bleeding.

Our take

Garlic gets a green light because studies suggest that garlic and garlic supplements may help lower low-density lipoprotein (LDL or "bad") cholesterol, and the supplements appear to be of low risk, except in individuals taking anti-clotting medications.

If you take garlic tablets, make sure they contain allicin, the active ingredient in garlic. Odor-free preparations may not include allicin.

What the research says

Several studies support garlic's use to lower cholesterol and reduce blood clot formation. A limited number of trials suggest that it may help relieve nausea during pregnancy. Preliminary studies indicate that garlic may help prevent cancer by interfering with the growth of malignant cells, as well as help prevent heart problems. The benefits appear to be modest.

Ginger

Ginger (*Zingiber officinale*) is an aromatic spice from Asia. The product you buy in grocery stores is the underground stem (rhizome) of the plant. It's also available as a powder, tablet, extract, tincture and oil.

Traditionally, ginger has been used to relieve nausea from pregnancy or motion sickness and to treat indigestion. It's not recommended for nausea during pregnancy if you have a history of bleeding disorders or miscarriages.

Our take

Ginger gets a green light because it's been shown to be somewhat effective in delaying motion sickness and in speeding recovery from it. It's generally considered safe when taken in small amounts and for a short term. High doses can cause abdominal discomfort.

Before taking ginger to prevent nausea associated with pregnancy, talk with your doctor.

What the research says

A limited number of studies suggest that ginger may help ease nausea from pregnancy when used for short periods.

Study results on the effectiveness of ginger to prevent nausea from motion sickness indicate it may be of benefit, but results have been mixed.

The benefits of ginger for treating nausea following anesthesia or chemotherapy is unclear.

Ginkgo

Ginkgo (*Ginkgo biloba*) is one of the oldest living species of tree. Its fan-shaped leaves as well as seeds have both been used in traditional medicine, but today most ginkgo products are made with extract prepared from the dried leaves.

The beneficial components of ginkgo are believed to be flavonoids, which have powerful antioxidant qualities, and terpenoids, which help improve circulation by dilating blood vessels and reducing the "stickiness" of platelets.

Ginkgo has been used to treat circulatory disorders and symptoms associated with reduced blood flow to the brain, particularly in older adults. These symptoms include short-term memory loss, dizziness, headache, ringing in the ears, depression and anxiety.

The herb is generally well tolerated but should be used cautiously if you're taking anti-clotting medication (including aspirin). You should also avoid the herb if you're taking a thiazide diuretic. Ginkgo may raise your blood pressure if used with this drug.

Our take

Studies have produced some encouraging results for the use of ginkgo as a treatment of certain circulation disorders and what are sometimes called cerebral insufficiencies — symptoms such as absent-mindedness and confusion — which may be associated with Alzheimer's disease. However, many questions remain unanswered, and the safety and effectiveness of ginkgo haven't always been proved. It's difficult to claim ginkgo as an unqualified "brain booster."

What the research says

Here's what some studies have found:

Claudication

A number of studies indicate that ginkgo causes small improvements in the symptoms of claudication, such as leg pain due to clogged arteries. However, ginkgo may not be as helpful for this condition as exercise or some prescription drugs.

Dementia

Many studies suggest that ginkgo benefits early-stage Alzheimer's disease and certain dementias, and it may be as helpful as drugs such as donepezil (Aricept). Much of this research is not well designed, and better studies are needed comparing ginkgo with standard prescription drug therapies.

Memory enhancement

Preliminary research shows slight improvements in memory and other brain functions in people with age-associated memory impairment, although some of the studies disagree. Overall, there's currently not enough evidence to recommend for or against this treatment. A recent, well-designed study reports that ginkgo did improve memory and concentration in older adults with no major memory problems.

Other

Studies indicate possible benefits of ginkgo in the treatment of depression and seasonal affective disorder, glaucoma, macular degeneration, tinnitus, sexual dysfunction and some premenstrual syndrome symptoms.

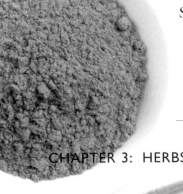

Ginseng

The term *ginseng* generally refers to two species of the plant, Asian ginseng (*Panax ginseng*) and American ginseng (*Panax quinquefolius*). Siberian ginseng (*Eleutherococcus senticosus*) is a different type of plant, and it doesn't contain the same active ingredients as Asian and American ginseng.

The gnarled, brown ginseng root is the part of the plant that's used in supplements. The root sometimes resembles a human body because of stringy offshoots that look like arms and legs. Due to that resemblance, practitioners of traditional Chinese medicine often considered the herb a cure-all for most human ills: allergies, asthma, appetite stimulant, bleeding disorders, breathing difficulties, cancer, dizziness, headache, insomnia, liver disease, heart palpitations, stroke, and many, many more.

It's best not to take ginseng for more than three months or to exceed the recommended maximum daily doses. Also don't take ginseng if you have uncontrolled high blood pressure, as the herb may raise blood pressure.

Our take

The sum total of evidence suggests that short-term use of ginseng may improve mental performance and that it produces few side effects when taken as directed, therefore we give it a green light. Never take ginseng for an extended period of time. More research is needed before specific recommendations regarding its use can be made.

More studies are also needed to determine ginseng's effectiveness against diabetes. Ginseng shouldn't be substituted for proven therapies.

What the research says

Here's what some studies have found:

Cancer

Several studies report that ginseng may reduce the risk of certain cancers, but all of this work was undertaken by the same research group and is considered preliminary.

Exercise performance

Athletes use ginseng to improve stamina, but it's unclear how much benefit it provides. Study results have been mixed.

Mental performance and mood

Studies report that ginseng can modestly improve the performance of thinking and learning tasks, based on measurements of reaction time, concentration and logic. It may also improve mood and enhance sleep. Although this evidence is promising, most studies have been small and not of the best design.

Type 2 diabetes

Several studies report that ginseng may lower blood sugar levels in people with type 2 diabetes, both at fasting states and after eating. The long-term effects of ginseng use are unknown, and more research is needed to determine what doses are safe and effective.

Well-being

Studies have examined the effects of ginseng to determine if it improves a sense of overall well-being in both healthy individuals and those who are ill. Results have been mixed.

Goldenseal

Goldenseal (*Hydrastis canadensis*) is a member of the buttercup family. It's commonly found in woodlands from Vermont to Arkansas and received its name from the gold scars on the base of the stem. Although once quite popular, its use has fallen out of favor.

The plant's underground stem (rhizome) contains an active ingredient called berberine, which may act as an antibiotic and mild laxative. Goldenseal is used to disinfect cuts and treat various inflammatory conditions, and it's prepared as a digestive aid. The herb is also combined with echinacea to treat upper respiratory tract infections.

Unfortunately, goldenseal can have serious side effects, especially when taken in high doses for long periods.

In the 1970s, a rumor circulated that people could use goldenseal to disguise the presence of illicit drugs in their bodies and thus avoid detection. Although this rumor is false, uncontrolled harvesting of the herb has helped to place it on the endangered species list.

Our take

Although goldenseal has demonstrated certain antibiotic and anti-inflammatory qualities, studies regarding the effectiveness and safety of this herb have been of poor quality. Goldenseal gets a red light because it can produce serious side effects if used for longer periods, and there's insufficient evidence that it works.

What the research says

Studies of goldenseal are limited and generally have been of poor quality:

Concealment of illicit drugs

Goldenseal gained a reputation for having the ability to interfere in the urine-testing process and mask illicit drugs, such as marijuana and cocaine, from detection. There's no reliable data to support this claim.

Infectious diarrhea

Several studies examined the use of goldenseal to treat infectious diarrhea. There are questions regarding the amount of active ingredient used and on whether this amount was significant enough to have an effect.

Upper respiratory tract infection

Goldenseal may be combined with echinacea to treat colds and upper respiratory tract infections. Although the ingredient berberine may possess certain antimicrobial qualities, its effect in humans needs more study.

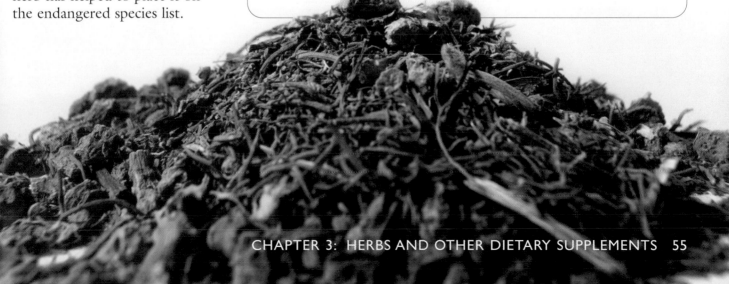

Green tea

Green tea is made from the dried leaves of *Camellia sinensis*, an evergreen shrub native to Southeast Asia. History dates its use in China as far back as 5,000 years ago. To this day, tea remains an integral part of daily life in many Asian societies, and consumption of green tea has become widespread throughout the world.

Processing the leaves of *Camellia sinensis* in different ways produces the different varieties of green tea, black tea and oolong tea. Tea contains polyphenols — compounds with strong antioxidant activity. Another active ingredient in tea is caffeine, which stimulates the nervous system and heart and acts as a diuretic.

People living in Asian countries, where green tea has been shown to have health benefits, have access to better quality green tea than do most Americans. Generally, the less processed the tea leaves are, the stronger the tea's antioxidant properties. To find the good stuff, check out Asian grocery stores or specialty tea shops.

Our take

Although all of the benefits of green tea still haven't been proved, it gets a green light because it does appear to have some medicinal qualities and it doesn't pose serious side effects. Drinking green tea possibly may help reduce the risk of various cancers. It's also linked to lower blood cholesterol and triglycerides. And it may help prevent or delay the onset of Parkinson's disease. Research on the tea's benefits is continuing, and we hope to know more in the near future.

What the research says

Here's what some studies have found:

Cancer prevention

Studies have examined the relationship between green tea drinking and the prevention of various cancers, including cancers of the digestive system, prostate, cervix and breast. Much of the research suggests green tea may possess cancer-protective qualities, but it's unclear whether other lifestyle factors may not play significant, if not greater, roles. Furthermore, large daily consumption of tea may be required for a relatively small benefit. Green tea doesn't appear to be of benefit in treating cancer.

Cardiovascular conditions

Several studies examined the effect of green tea on cardiovascular health. Results suggest that the tea may improve cholesterol levels and reduce risk of stroke, heart attack and atherosclerosis. The Food and Drug Administration has stated that there's no credible scientific evidence to back these claims.

Longevity

A 2006 study involving 40,000 people in Japan found the more green tea people drank, the longer they lived. Cardiovascular disease was significantly less common among those who drink more than five cups a day.

Obesity

Small trials have looked at the association between green tea consumption and weight loss or maintenance. More research is necessary to make any recommendation.

Hawthorn

Hawthorn (multiple *crataegus* species) is a thorny shrub from the rose family. Historically, the fruit was used in traditional medicine, but today extracts from the flowers and leaves are more common.

It's a popular alternative medicine for cardiovascular health. Active ingredients include flavonoids, which are known to help dilate blood vessels, improve blood flow and increase heart rate. Other ingredients in hawthorn have powerful antioxidant effects.

 Our take

Although hawthorn appears to have some positive benefits regarding cardiovascular health, not enough is known about its effectiveness and safety. Don't self-medicate with hawthorn. If you have a heart condition, talk with your doctor before taking the herb.

What the research says

Results from multiple studies indicate that hawthorn may be beneficial in the treatment of congestive heart failure. However, there's insufficient evidence regarding its effectiveness in treating coronary artery disease, angina and other cardiovascular disorders.

Hoodia

Hoodia (*Hoodia gordonii*) is a cactus native to the Kalahari Desert in southern Africa. The native San people have been known to eat hoodia to ward off hunger and thirst during long hunts.

The active ingredient has been identified as P57. This compound is believed to stimulate the hypothalamus, a portion of the brain's interior that turns off hunger signals. You end up thinking you're full even if you haven't eaten. This quality has made hoodia a popular ingredient in weight-loss products.

 Our take

There's still too much that's unknown about hoodia to recommend its use. More research is needed to establish its potential effectiveness and long-term safety as an appetite suppressant. In addition, unregulated products claiming to contain hoodia may have little or none of the active ingredient.

What the research says

To date, no objective, long-term studies have been undertaken to demonstrate the effectiveness and safety of hoodia as an appetite suppressant. One small study — sponsored by a supplement manufacturer — suggests that the herb affects the part of the brain that controls hunger.

Kava

Kava comes from a pepper plant called *Piper methysticum* that's native to the South Pacific islands. The root of the plant is a source of extracts and powder. Kava is also commonly consumed as a beverage.

The active ingredient in kava acts as a sedative and a muscle relaxant. Therefore, it became popular as a stress and anxiety reliever. Some people use it to relieve insomnia.

Because of its sedating effects, kava should never be taken before driving or operating heavy machinery. And it shouldn't be mixed with alcohol or other sedatives.

Our take

Kava appeared to be a promising treatment for stress and anxiety, but reports of serious liver problems — even with short-term use — caused the herb to lose its luster. The damage is associated with the concentrated form of kava. It's still not clear if kava beverages carry a similar risk. Regardless, avoid kava until more information is available.

What the research says

Numerous well-conducted studies have found kava to be at least moderately effective in the treatment of anxiety. In fact, kava may be as effective as certain prescribed medications. However, reports of severe liver damage linked to its use have caused several European countries to pull it off the market. The Food and Drug Administration has issued warnings but not banned sales.

Mangosteen

Mangosteen (*Garcinia mangostana*) is a tropical fruit native to Southeast Asia. The fruit is tangerine-sized with a hard purple rind that encases an edible white pulp. It's not a relative of the mango fruit.

Mangosteen contains many active plant chemicals (phytochemicals) including xanthones, which are antioxidants thought to boost the immune system. No adverse side effects have been reported.

Because it's not readily available in the United States, products made with mangosteen are generally expensive.

Our take

Mangosteen shows possible promise as an immune system booster, helping your body to fight off germs and infection. But it lacks good quality evidence demonstrating that either the fruit or its juice is an effective treatment. At this time, don't expect much beyond the nutritional benefit of its fruit.

What the research says

Mangosteen has been credited with anti-allergy, antibacterial, antifungal, antihistamine and anti-inflammatory qualities. It's also been touted as a cancer treatment. To date, though, there aren't any high-quality human trials under way that support its effectiveness or determine its safety, with either short-term or long-term use.

Milk thistle

Milk thistle (*Silybum marianum*) is a member of the aster family and named from the white veins on its spiked, variegated leaves. It was commonly used in ancient Greece and Rome to treat disorders of the liver and gallbladder.

The active ingredient in milk thistle is silymarin, which is extracted from the plant's seeds. This flavonoid is believed to have antioxidant qualities. Milk thistle is considered safe to use within recommended amounts, and it typically doesn't produce any side effects.

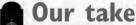

Our take

Milk thistle gets a green light because its active ingredients appear to protect the liver and block or remove harmful substances from the organ. It has the potential to be developed into a prescription drug. More extensive research is still needed to determine the herb's efficacy and also to find out if it produces any negative long-term effects.

What the research says

Multiple studies suggest that milk thistle improves organ function in people with cirrhosis, a chronic liver disease. Research also indicates that the herb is beneficial in the treatment of chronic hepatitis brought on by viruses or alcohol use. Although promising, better research is necessary before specific recommendations can be made.

Mistletoe

Mistletoe (*Viscum album*) was a sacred herb in Celtic traditions and considered a "cure-all." The two major types of mistletoe are the European and American varieties, which are quite different plants.

Mistletoe has been used in Europe as an anti-cancer therapy. It's not an accepted treatment in the United States.

Mistletoe extracts are prescription drugs given by injection. It's important to note that you should never eat any part of the plant or drink the extract because mistletoe is poisonous.

Our take

In Germany, it's common for people with cancer to take mistletoe in addition to receiving chemotherapy or radiation. Despite its widespread acceptance in Europe, the herb lacks good data to back up its effectiveness and safety. While mistletoe may hold some promise as a cancer treatment, better research is needed before we feel comfortable recommending its use.

What the research says

An extensive body of literature exists regarding use of mistletoe to treat cancer, but the individual studies have been small or of poor design. Therefore, not enough is known about the herb. Although mistletoe extract has shown the ability to stimulate the immune system, there's no evidence that this bolstered immunity prevents or kills cancer cells.

Noni juice

Noni (*Morinda citrifolia*) is a small tree native to the Pacific Islands and Polynesia. It's also known as the Indian mulberry.

The juice from the foul-smelling, bitter-tasting noni fruit is used to treat a wide range of conditions, including arthritis, diabetes, high blood pressure, pain, diarrhea, cancer, AIDS, multiple sclerosis and bad breath. These claims are usually based on testimonials, often from the people who are attempting to sell noni products.

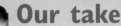
Our take
When a product is advertised to treat almost every ailment, that's generally a good indication there's more "hype" than "help" at play. There's no convincing evidence that noni juice has any beneficial effect on your health. Orange juice and apple juice contain more antioxidants than does the noni fruit.

What the research says
At least one clinical trial involving noni juice is under way — this one to study the effects of noni juice on people in the advanced stages of cancer. Some studies show that noni juice has antioxidant qualities, but likely no more than almost any other type of fruit. Despite the claims, there's no evidence that noni juice reduces cholesterol.

Passionflower

Passionflower (*Passiflora incarnata*) is a woody vine native to North America, but today it's mainly grown throughout Europe.

American Indians used the herb as a mild sedative. It has been used in traditional medicine for anxiety, insomnia, restlessness and any conditions with possible emotional or psychological origins.

Generally, passionflower is considered safe when used as a flavoring or taken within recommended amounts. In Europe, it's combined with other herbs as an over-the-counter sedative.

Our take
As a folk medicine, passionflower has a long history and though it lacks good evidence as to its effectiveness, small studies have shown it may reduce anxiety. The herb is generally considered safe to use, as long as you take it according to directions. Keep in mind that because it's a sedative it can cause drowsiness, and in some cases may cause a rapid heart rate or nausea.

What the research says
Passionflower lacks quality clinical trials to show that it effectively treats anxiety or restlessness. Further complicating matters is the fact that passionflower is often combined with hawthorn and valerian in commercial products, making it difficult to distinguish the unique qualities of each herb.

Among the studies that have been done, the herb generally hasn't been found to cause serious side effects.

Peppermint

Besides being a popular flavoring, peppermint (*Mentha x piperita*) has a long history of use for digestive symptoms such as indigestion, nausea, cramps and diarrhea, as well as for colds and headaches.

The main active ingredient is the phytochemical menthol, which helps relax stomach muscles and improve the flow of bile, allowing food to pass through the stomach faster. Peppermint also has a soothing effect on skin irritations. The herb is generally considered safe for use with few side effects.

Our take

Peppermint has some benefits in treating certain digestive disorders such as irritable bowel syndrome and possibly heartburn. However, its muscle-relaxing qualities could worsen heartburn symptoms associated with gastroesophageal reflux disease (GERD), so take it under a doctor's supervision. There's insufficient evidence that peppermint can treat colds, nasal congestion and tension headaches.

What the research says

Multiple trials suggest that the symptoms of irritable bowel syndrome can improve significantly with enteric-coated peppermint capsules. There's also preliminary evidence that a combination of peppermint oil and caraway oil can alleviate symptoms of heartburn (dyspepsia). More research involving larger, better designed studies is needed to fully determine its effectiveness.

Policosanol

Policosanol is a mixture of alcohol-based compounds derived from sugar cane or beeswax. It's used to protect against heart disease, by lowering cholesterol levels, and is taken to reduce the risk of blood clots.

It's unknown what the active ingredient in policosanol is or how it works, but the supplement is generally safe and well tolerated.

Most studies of policosanol have taken place in Cuba using Cuban sugar cane. Although more than 25 countries currently use policosanol, products are not always readily available in the United States.

Our take

Initial studies on the benefits of policosanol all were done in Cuba — where sugar cane is grown — and all of the studies were positive. More recent studies done outside of Cuba haven't produced the same benefits. This draws into question the plant's ability to reduce cholesterol, along with other heart-health claims. It likely won't harm you to give policosanol a try, but you could be wasting your money.

What the research says

A number of studies have demonstrated that policosanol can reduce low-density lipoprotein (LDL or "bad") cholesterol and triglyceride levels and raise high-density lipoprotein (HDL or "good") cholesterol levels. However, two recent studies found the product ineffective. There are also questions regarding optimal dose and long-term safety. Other studies have suggested that the plant may be effective in preventing blood from clotting.

Pycnogenol

Pycnogenol is a compound derived from the bark of the maritime pine (*Pinus pinaster*), native to the coast of southern France.

The supplement has antioxidant qualities similar to those of green tea and grape seed. Antioxidants help neutralize highly reactive molecules known as free radicals that can damage your body's cells.

Pycnogenol is generally considered safe to use at recommended doses, with no significant side effects.

Our take

Pycnogenol may have a future role as an antioxidant. It should be noted, though, that pycnogenol probably contains nothing that can't be gained from a diet rich in vegetables and fruits. Because the name is trademarked and patented to a single company, pycnogenol is likely to be a more expensive option.

What the research says

Pycnogenol has been used as an antioxidant and to treat diabetes, high cholesterol, blood clotting, retinopathy and attention-deficit hyperactivity disorder (ADHD). However, long-term, well-designed studies are yet to be undertaken. At this time, not a lot is known about how it works or what should be a standardized dose.

Red yeast rice

Red yeast rice is the product of yeast (*Monascus purpureus*) grown on white rice. The powdered yeast-rice mixture is a dietary staple in many parts of Asia and has been used in traditional Chinese medicine, primarily for heart problems.

Red yeast rice contains several compounds that appear to lower cholesterol levels. One of the compounds is monacolin K, the same ingredient as in the prescription cholesterol drug lovastatin (Mevacor). This has led to a legal and industrial dispute as to whether red yeast rice should be considered a drug or a dietary supplement.

Our take

Red yeast rice is capable of lowering blood cholesterol levels and while the supplement is generally considered safe, it also carries the same potential side effects as statin cholesterol drugs. The only advantage of taking red yeast rice in place of a statin drug may be the cheaper cost. However, with a supplement, there's less assurance regarding quality and how much active ingredient is actually in the product you buy.

What the research says

A number of studies indicate that red yeast rice can lower your total blood cholesterol level, your low-density lipoprotein (LDL or "bad") cholesterol level and your triglyceride level.

Cholestin was a well-known, nonprescription brand of red yeast rice extract until the Food and Drug Administration ruled it was a drug and attempted to block sales. The manufacturer has since reformulated Cholestin without the extract.

Saw palmetto

Saw palmetto (*Serenoa repens*) is a fan palm that thrives in the United States' warm southeastern climate. The dark purple berries were a staple food of American Indians and also used as an expectorant and antiseptic.

There are many products on the market today containing saw palmetto, frequently in combination with other ingredients. In Europe, saw palmetto is used to treat the symptoms of benign prostatic hyperplasia (BPH) — an enlarged prostate. Although saw palmetto is a popular treatment for BPH in the United States, it's not considered a standard treatment.

Our take

Saw palmetto seemed to be an effective treatment for managing symptoms of an enlarged prostate, but a recent study stole some of its luster. This isn't to say that the herb isn't effective, but it does suggest the need for more research to better understand its benefits.

Saw palmetto is generally safe when used as directed and side effects are rare, but you shouldn't use it if you have a bleeding problem. If you have urinary symptoms, don't self-diagnose your condition. Talk to your doctor before trying saw palmetto.

What the research says

A number of studies have suggested that saw palmetto can increase urine flow, diminish inflammation, reduce nighttime urination and improve the overall quality of life for individuals dealing with an enlarged prostate. However — contrary to previous studies — a recent trial found no significant benefits in the use of saw palmetto to treat enlarged prostate, putting the herb's medicinal abilities into question.

It's not clear if the herb actually reduces the size of the prostate or just improves symptoms. Older studies suggest that in some individuals saw palmetto may be as effective as the anti-androgenic drug finasteride (Proscar).

'Herbal viagras' — Are they safe?

Prescription medications such as sildenafil (Viagra) treat erectile dysfunction by increasing blood flow to the penis when a man is sexually aroused. Some herbal products marketed as "natural versions" of these stimulants contain substances that improve blood flow, but are not as specific for blood vessels in the penis as are the prescription drugs. As a result, these herbal remedies may cause generalized low blood pressure and restrict blood flow to vital organs.

The Food and Drug Administration recently warned of several dietary supplements sold to treat erectile dysfunction and promote sexual enhancement as unapproved, illegal and risky because they contain potentially harmful drugs that aren't included on the product label. These include the supplements Actra-Rx, 4Everon, Libidus, Nasutra, Neophase, Vigor-25 and Zimaxx. The herb ginseng is widely believed to enhance sexual performance but, lacking significant quality control, it's often difficult to know what kind of product you're getting. Another popular herb called yohimbe can be dangerous if used in excessive amounts.

The bottom line: If you have erectile dysfunction, see your doctor to discuss proven treatment options.

Soy

Soy (*Glycine max*) is a member of the pea family and native to southeastern Asia. The soybean has been a dietary staple of Asian countries for thousands of years. Fermentation techniques allow soy to be prepared in more easily digestible forms such as tempe, miso, tofu and tamari (soy) sauce.

Active ingredients in soy include isoflavones, weak forms of estrogen that mimic your own naturally occurring estrogen. For that reason, isoflavones are also known as phytoestrogens. How beneficial they are to your body is still being studied.

Interestingly — despite its broad popularity — no one has thoroughly tested the safety and effectiveness of soy as a supplement. Therefore, much about it is still uncertain.

Our take

Diets high in soy foods do have health benefits. For example, soy is a great source of dietary protein minus all of the fat and cholesterol found in meat. Soy also provides fiber, vitamins and minerals. But claims that soy can reduce blood cholesterol levels are uncertain.

Little is known about soy supplements. Although they appear to be safe, use them under your doctor's supervision and with the knowledge that they may be of limited benefit.

What the research says

Here's what some of the research suggests:

Cancer

A few studies attempted to determine the impact of a soy-based diet on hormone-related cancers such as breast, colon and endometrial cancers. So far, there are more questions than there are answers, and more extensive study is needed.

Cardiovascular disease

Studies suggest that soy doesn't affect long-term cardiovascular outcomes such as heart attack or stroke.

High cholesterol

Conventional wisdom was that adding soy to your diet produced a moderate decrease in cholesterol levels. This view changed after the American Heart Association, following an extensive review of research, concluded that soy-based foods don't significantly lower cholesterol. In addition, the reduction in low-density lipoprotein (LDL or "bad") cholesterol came from eating large amounts of soy, not the relatively small amounts found in many food products.

Menopausal symptoms

Research has examined the effects of soy products containing isoflavones on the reduction of menopausal symptoms such as hot flashes. Although the results so far have been mixed, evidence overall suggests some benefit.

St. John's wort

St. John's wort (*Hypericum perforatum*) is a flowering shrub that gets its name from the fact that it's often in full bloom on the traditional date of the birthday of the biblical John the Baptist. It has a long history as a treatment for depression, anxiety, insomnia and nervous disorders. It's also prepared as a salve for wounds and burns.

The flowers and leaves contain active ingredients such as hyperforin. But there are other, still unidentified but very active, components in the plant. It's available in tablet, powder and liquid form.

Although St. John's wort is believed to be safe for general use, some of its active compounds don't mix well with prescription drugs and other supplements. These include antidepressant medications, birth control pills, anticoagulant drugs, certain asthma medications and steroids.

Our take

St. John's wort is effective in treating mild to moderate depression and it's relatively safe. It's drawback — and the reason we give it a yellow light instead of a green — is that it interacts with many medications and has caused serious side effects. You shouldn't take St. John's wort if you take prescription medications. It's also important to talk to your doctor before taking St. John's wort. If you have a more severe form of depression, you may need a stronger medication.

What the research says

Studies have generally focused on depression and anxiety:

Anxiety

Studies have examined the effectiveness of St. John's wort on symptoms of anxiety. In one case, St. John's wort was combined with the herb valerian. At this time, there's not enough evidence to make a recommendation.

Depression

Several studies support the therapeutic benefit of St. John's wort in treating mild to moderate depression. It's been shown to be as effective as some prescription antidepressants and with fewer side effects. Two studies reported no benefits for major depression. The greatest concern with using St. John's wort is the potential for serious interactions with various types of prescription drugs.

Choosing the right brand

With so many manufacturers of supplements to choose from, how do you know what's a good brand — and that the product actually contains what it says it does? Here are some suggestions:

- **Look for standardized supplements.** The U.S. Pharmacopeia's USP Dietary Supplement Verified seal on the label indicates the product has met certain manufacturing standards. Other groups that certify supplements include ConsumerLab.com, *Good Housekeeping* and NSF International. Although each group takes a slightly different approach, the goal of each is to certify the product meets a certain standard.

- **Look for a large, recognizable manufacturer.** While this isn't a guarantee that the product contains exactly what it says it does, chances are better that a well-known company with a good reputation will make the effort to produce a quality product.

- **Be cautious about supplements manufactured outside the United States.** Many European herbs and other dietary supplements are highly regulated and standardized. But toxic ingredients and prescription drugs have been found in some supplements manufactured in other countries.

Stinging nettle

The leaves and stem of stinging nettle (*Urtica dioica*) are covered with tiny hairs containing histamine, an irritating chemical when it comes in contact with the skin. The plant is often used for treating enlarged prostate, often in combination with saw palmetto. It's also used to treat allergic rhinitis, arthritis and joint pain, and insect bites.

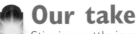 **Our take**

Stinging nettle is generally regarded as safe to use. It's even consumed as a vegetable or made into tea. But how effective it is in treating conditions such as enlarged prostate is uncertain.

What the research says

Several studies suggest that stinging nettle moderately improves symptoms of enlarged prostate. Stinging nettle also may have certain anti-inflammatory qualities for treating joint pain. In both cases, more research is needed.

Tea tree oil

The tea tree (*Melaleuca alternifolia*) is native to Australia. Distillation of its leaves produces an oil believed to have antiseptic qualities and used to treat infections and wounds.

Avoid taking tea tree oil orally as there are reports of severe toxic reactions, including rash, abdominal pain and diarrhea.

Our take

Tea tree oil is a common ingredient in shampoos and acne medications, but there's little information from human studies as to its effectiveness as an antiseptic.

What the research says

Laboratory tests indicate that tea tree oil has certain antimicrobial qualities that may be useful for treating fungal infections, acne and allergic skin reactions. Additional testing in humans is the next step in determining its effectiveness.

Valerian

Valerian (*Valeriana officinalis*) is a tall, flowering grassland plant that has long been used as a tranquilizer and to treat insomnia, anxiety and stress.

Products such as teas are made from the plant's roots, although the active ingredient is not identified. It's generally considered safe to use, although it may cause headaches.

Our take

Valerian appears to be beneficial for insomnia and anxiety and is generally safe at recommended doses. Don't take valerian for more than a few weeks at a time.

What the research says

Results from several small or short-term studies indicate that valerian may help you fall asleep and may improve sleep quality. Valerian may also reduce the symptoms of anxiety but this requires further research.

Vitamins

Vitamin B-3 (niacin)

Vitamin B-3 (niacin) is one of the eight B complex vitamins that help the body convert food to energy. Niacin also helps improve blood circulation and cholesterol levels.

Food sources of niacin include lean meats, poultry, fish, peanuts and brewer's yeast. The recommended daily intake of niacin is 16 milligrams (mg) for men and 14 mg for women.

Seek your doctor's advice before taking a niacin supplement if you have diabetes, gallbladder or liver disease, or glaucoma.

Our take

Niacin may be used to help improve your cholesterol levels, but this should only be done under a doctor's supervision. Cholesterol-lowering effects typically require large doses (usually greater than 1,000 milligrams per day). In this respect, niacin should be considered a prescribed medication and not a vitamin.

What the research says

Niacin in high doses can reduce low-density lipoprotein (LDL or "bad") cholesterol and triglycerides and raise high-density lipoprotein (HDL or "good") cholesterol. Studies show that niacin may also slow the development of atherosclerosis when used with other cholesterol-lowering drugs, diet and exercise. A recent study suggests that niacin may help protect against Alzheimer's disease and age-related mental decline.

Vitamin B-6

Vitamin B-6 (pyridoxine) is an important vitamin for normal brain development and for keeping the nervous system and immune system healthy.

Food sources of vitamin B-6 include poultry, fish, potatoes, lentils, soybeans, whole-grain products, nuts, seeds, carrots and bananas. It can also be taken as a supplement.

There are medications, including certain antibiotics and birth control pills, that interfere with the metabolism of vitamin B-6, possibly causing a vitamin deficiency.

Our take

Vitamin B-6 supplements are effective for treating a hereditary form of anemia and for preventing an adverse reaction to the antibiotic cycloserine. They should be taken under medical supervision.

What the research says

Vitamin B-6 has been shown to work together with vitamins B-9 and B 12 to control blood levels of homocysteine. Elevated levels of homocysteine increase your risk of heart attack or stroke.

More research is required of vitamin B-6 as a remedy for premenstrual syndrome (PMS) and carpal tunnel syndrome. The large doses required for treatment can be associated with side effects.

Vitamin B-9 (folate or folic acid)

Vitamin B-9, also called folate, occurs naturally in certain foods. Folic acid is the synthetic form of folate. This vitamin is important in red blood cell formation and for healthy cell growth and function. It's also important for the developing fetus during pregnancy.

Food sources of folate include citrus juices and fruits, beans, nuts, seeds, dark green leafy vegetables and fortified grain products. Folic acid is found in supplements and in fortified breads and cereals.

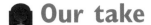

Our take

There's solid evidence that folate or folic acid can prevent neural tube birth defects such as spina bifida, heart disease and possibly some cancers. If you don't get adequate folate in your diet, consider taking a folic acid supplement or multivitamin. Women planning to become pregnant should take 400 micrograms of folic acid daily.

What the research says

Folic acid has been shown to work together with vitamins B-6 and B-12 to control elevated blood levels of homocysteine, reducing your risk of heart attack and stroke. Studies indicate that folate can help prevent anemia during pregnancy and reduce the risk of birth defects. Preliminary results suggest that folate may reduce the risk of breast, cervical and pancreatic cancer.

Vitamin B-12

Vitamin B-12 (cobalamin) plays essential roles in red blood cell formation, cell metabolism, nerve function and production of DNA.

Sources of vitamin B-12 are animal foods, including meat, poultry, fish, shellfish, eggs and dairy products. Many breakfast cereals are vitamin fortified.

Your body is capable of storing several years' worth of vitamin B-12, so a deficiency is rare. However, vegetarians who completely eliminate meat from their diets are prone to a deficiency of this vitamin.

Our take

It's essential to get sufficient amounts of vitamin B-12 because of its importance to almost every body system. Most children and adults in the United States consume recommended amounts of vitamin B-12. Generally, older adults are at a greater risk of developing a deficiency. Supplements are important for vegetarians, as plant foods don't contain vitamin B-12.

What the research says

Studies show that a deficiency of vitamin B-12 can produce abnormal neurological and psychiatric symptoms, including anemia, fatigue, muscle weakness, dementia and mood disturbances.

Preliminary research reveals possibilities for vitamin B-12, in combination with other ingredients, for treating cardiovascular disease, high cholesterol, breast cancer and Alzheimer's disease.

Vitamin C

Vitamin C (ascorbic acid) is necessary for the development of healthy bones and muscles, and it's vital in the healing process. Vitamin C also has strong antioxidant properties.

The human body doesn't produce vitamin C, so it's necessary to include it in your diet. Food sources include citrus fruits, berries, tomatoes, peppers, broccoli and spinach. Supplements come as tablets, capsules and chewables.

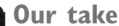

Our take

Vitamin C is important to your physical health and meeting the recommended dietary allowance (75 mg to 90 mg for adults) is considered essential. Few of the many purported medical uses of vitamin C supplements — to treat asthma, diabetes and cancer — have been proved in scientific studies. Using supplements to treat the common cold remains controversial; however, there's nothing else better and preliminary evidence suggests the supplements may be beneficial.

What the research says

Many studies have examined the effect of vitamin C consumption on the prevention and treatment of the common cold. Most have failed to show significant benefits but research is ongoing.

Vitamin C doesn't appear to lower cholesterol or prevent stroke. Large population studies have associated high vitamin C intake with reduced risk of cancer, but this requires further study.

Vitamin D

Your body manufactures vitamin D when direct sunlight converts a chemical in your skin into an active form of the vitamin (calciferol). Vitamin D is necessary for building and maintaining healthy bones. That's because calcium, the primary component of bone, can only be absorbed by your body when vitamin D is present.

You can also get vitamin D from certain dietary sources, including fortified milk, fortified cereal and fatty fish such as salmon, mackerel and sardines.

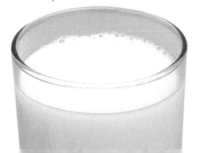

Our take

There's a lot of interest in vitamin D, and it's possible we may see a change in recommendations. The current recommended dietary allowance for vitamin D is 200 international units (IU) for people ages 19 to 49 years, 400 IU for people ages 50 to 70 years, and 600 IU for those older than 70. If you don't get adequate vitamin D from your diet or being outside, supplements may be necessary. But be aware that high doses of vitamin D (more than 1,000 IU) can be harmful.

What the research says

Studies show that people with adequate amounts of vitamin D and calcium in their diets can prevent or slow osteoporosis and reduce the number of fractures. Research also suggests that vitamin D may reduce the risk of rheumatoid arthritis, multiple sclerosis and certain cancers. A vitamin D deficiency is associated with osteomalacia and muscle pain.

Vitamin E

Vitamin E has antioxidant properties, which protect body tissues from damage caused by free radicals — unstable molecules associated with degenerative processes brought on by aging and chronic disease. Vitamin E also protects red blood cells and is important in reproduction.

Vitamin E exists in eight different forms, and the most active form — typically found in supplements — is known as alpha-tocopherol. Food sources of vitamin E include vegetable oils, wheat germ, whole-grain products, avocados, green leafy vegetables and nuts, especially almonds.

For years, vitamin E was thought to offer protection against such conditions as heart disease, cancer, Alzheimer's disease and cataracts. As a result, many people began taking supplements in megadoses. But a recent analysis of clinical trials found more was not necessarily better when it came to this vitamin. High daily intake may pose health risks and should be avoided. The harm or benefits of taking lower doses remains uncertain.

The recommended dietary allowance is 22 international units (IU) a day from dietary sources or 33 IU from supplements.

Our take

It's known that getting plenty of vitamin E in your diet is good for you. Therefore, the belief was that vitamin E supplements would be beneficial, too. However, studies involving people who took alpha-tocopherol vitamin E supplements have produced negative results. This has led researchers to question if other forms of vitamin E might be better than alpha-tocopherol, including a "mixed" vitamin E supplement, which contains all eight forms. We don't know the answer yet. Or, it may be that you can't beat mother nature, and there aren't any supplements that provide the benefits of natural vitamin E in foods.

If you do decide to take a vitamin E supplement, don't take more than 400 International Units (IU) daily, unless otherwise directed by your doctor.

What the research says

Here's what studies have found:

Cancer

There's no scientific evidence that vitamin E is effective treatment for any type of cancer. High-dose antioxidants may reduce the effects of chemotherapy and radiation therapy.

Cardiovascular disease

Although research results conflict, recent studies show no benefits in the prevention of cardiovascular disease.

Dementia

Vitamin E has been evaluated for the prevention of dementia, but so far the evidence has been inconclusive.

High doses

An analysis of previous studies found that people who consumed at least 400 IU of vitamin E daily for at least a year could be at an increased risk of premature death. It should be noted that many of the study participants had chronic illnesses. And in many of the trials, the participants took supplements containing multiple antioxidants, masking the specific role played by vitamin E.

Vision

Studies of the effects of vitamin E on cataracts and macular degeneration have been inconclusive.

Multivitamins: Do you need one?

The best way to get your vitamins and minerals is through a balanced diet. However, there are times when a supplement containing a variety of vitamins and minerals — commonly referred to as a multivitamin pill — may be appropriate.

If you don't eat well — you don't eat the recommended servings of fruits, vegetables and other healthy foods — you may benefit from a vitamin and mineral supplement. In addition, if you have to limit your diet because of food allergies or intolerance to certain foods, a supplement may be appropriate. Multivitamins are also recommended for strict vegetarians who eat no animal products. These individuals may not get enough vitamin B-12, zinc, iron and calcium.

If you're over age 65, there are a variety of reasons why you may not get the nutrients you need. A multivitamin may make more sense than taking single-nutrient pills.

It's generally recommended that pregnant or breast-feeding women take additional vitamins, but you should discuss what to take with your doctor.

What to watch for

Consider these points when choosing a multivitamin:
- **Iron.** Although supplemental iron is advised during pregnancy and for iron deficiency anemia, too much iron can be toxic. For men and post-menopausal women, it's probably wise to take a pill with little or no iron — 8 milligrams (mg) a day or less. "Senior formulas" generally have less iron.

- **Vitamin B-6 (pyridoxine).** Adequate levels of this vitamin may help lower blood homocysteine, a possible risk factor for heart attack, and improve immune system function. Older adults who lack variety in their diets may not get enough vitamin B-6, so a multivitamin that contains about 2 mg is often a good idea. Avoid excessive doses. Too much vitamin B-6 can result in nerve damage to the arms and legs, which is usually reversible when supplementation is stopped.

- **Vitamin B-12 (cobalamin).** Adequate levels of this vitamin may reduce your risk of anemia, cardiovascular disease and stroke. Older adults often don't absorb this vitamin well. A multivitamin with at least 2 micrograms (mcg) may help.

- **Vitamin D.** This vitamin helps the body absorb calcium and is essential in maintaining bone strength and bone density. Many older adults don't get regular exposure to sunlight and have trouble absorbing vitamin D, so taking a multivitamin with 400 to 600 international units (IU) will likely help improve bone health.

- **Vitamin E.** A recent review of studies indicates that taking daily vitamin E supplements of 400 IU or more — and possibly as low as 150 IU — may pose health risks. Talk with your doctor before taking vitamin E supplements.

5 things you should know

1. Multivitamins don't need to cost much. Most generic products and store brands are fine.

2. Look for a third-party verification on the label, such as USPV or NFS. This means the product has been tested in a laboratory and meets standards of quality.

3. Look for a multivitamin that contains a wide variety of vitamins and minerals in the appropriate amounts, usually 100 percent of the Daily Value (DV). Check the contents to make sure you're not getting too much of any nutrient, which can be harmful. In most cases, if the tablet doesn't exceed 100 percent of the DV, it's considered safe.

4. Take your multivitamin with food. If it contains iron, don't take a calcium supplement at the same time, since iron interferes with calcium absorption.

5. Claims such as "stress formula," "high potency," "natural" or "slow release" are often just marketing ploys and only add to the price.

Calcium

Calcium is the most abundant mineral in the human body. In addition to the support it provides to your skeleton, calcium is also needed for your heart, muscles and nerves to function properly. Your body also has built-in safeguards to maintain an adequate amount of calcium in your bloodstream.

Contrary to popular belief, need for the mineral actually increases with age. That's because the human body requires constant replenishment and, with age, the body becomes less efficient at absorbing calcium from the diet. For women, a drop in estrogen levels at menopause further reduces calcium absorption. In addition, some older adults tend to eat fewer dietary products that contain calcium.

Dietary sources of calcium include dairy products such as milk, cheese and yogurt, calcium-fortified cereals and juice, greens (spinach, bok choy, collards, kale, turnip), broccoli, green soybeans (edamame), and fish that are eaten with their bones (salmon, sardines).

Many people simply don't get enough calcium in their diets. American adults typically eat less than 600 milligrams (mg) daily, but the recommended daily intake ranges from 1,000 to 1,200 mg or more.

Our take

Dietary sources of calcium may be better for you than supplements because the foods contain other important nutrients as well. But if you struggle to get enough calcium in your diet, taking a supplement is fine. Calcium supplements are generally safe.

What the research says

Here's what some studies have found:

Calcium deficiency

Calcium supplements can ease the symptoms of mineral deficiency in people who don't get adequate amounts of the vitamin. A deficiency can cause low blood calcium levels, muscle spasms and low levels of parathyroid hormone.

High blood pressure

Calcium intake at normal recommended levels may help prevent or treat symptoms of moderate hypertension.

Osteoporosis

High calcium intake, through the use of supplements, helps reduce the loss of bone density in older adults and postmenopausal women, reducing the risk of osteoporosis. In people who have osteoporosis, calcium and vitamin D taken in combination with prescribed medications may be beneficial.

Premenstrual syndrome

Calcium intake at recommended levels may reduce some of the symptoms of premenstrual syndrome (PMS).

Chromium

Chromium is a trace mineral — trace meaning that, although essential, it's needed by the body in only small amounts. Dietary sources of chromium include whole grains, seafood, green beans, broccoli, potatoes and peanuts.

Although the exact role played by chromium isn't fully understood, it appears to assist in the cellular response to the hormone insulin. Because of this function, chromium is often associated with the treatment of diabetes and weight-loss products.

 Our take

Although many American diets are low in chromium, it's rare to have a chromium deficiency. And be aware that diabetes is not a chromium-deficient disease. It's best to eat a balanced diet that includes sources of chromium and take supplements only under a doctor's supervision.

What the research says

Chromium interacts with insulin, so it's natural to think that supplements would have a positive impact on diabetes. Research results so far have been mixed. There's also no scientific evidence that chromium supplements have any benefit for weight loss. Although studies suggest that supplements may help control cholesterol levels, there may be better ways to accomplish this.

Iron

Iron plays an essential role in delivering oxygen to the body via the bloodstream. It also has many muscular and metabolic functions.

Dietary sources of iron include meat, seafood, poultry, whole grains, beans, peas and dark green leafy vegetables. The recommended dietary allowance for adult males and most women over 50 is 8 milligrams (mg). Women of childbearing years should have 18 mg daily.

Lack of iron leads to anemia and reduces your resistance to infection. Too much iron can cause hemochromatosis, which can lead to diabetes and liver damage.

 Our take

For most healthy men and postmenopausal women, iron deficiency is rare. To get enough iron, eat a balanced diet containing iron-rich foods. Women of childbearing age and people with conditions that cause internal bleeding, such as ulcers, may require iron supplements. Dieters, athletes and vegetarians who don't consume animal products also may require higher amounts of dietary iron.

What the research says

Studies show that iron supplements can prevent or treat iron deficiency anemia, a condition where there are too few red blood cells to adequately carry oxygen to the body. This can result from too little iron in the diet. Research also has demonstrated that iron supplements may benefit women during menstruation or pregnancy.

Magnesium

Magnesium is involved in many biochemical reactions in the body, helping to maintain normal heart rhythm, immune system and muscle function.

Dietary sources of magnesium include legumes, whole grains, dark green leafy vegetables and nuts. Supplements combine the mineral with another substance, for example magnesium citrate or magnesium gluconate. Your doctor may recommend supplements if necessary levels of magnesium can't be achieved through your daily diet.

Our take

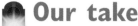

It's uncommon for Americans to experience a deficiency in magnesium. Supplements are generally necessary only when a health problem or drug interaction causes excessive magnesium loss or limits absorption.

When taken with food, magnesium supplements are less likely to cause side effects such as diarrhea, nausea and abdominal cramps.

What the research says

Low magnesium levels are linked with a variety of conditions, including high blood pressure, heart disease, osteoporosis and poorly controlled diabetes. Use of certain medications, such as diuretics, and certain antibiotics also may affect magnesium levels. Studies suggest supplements may reduce some symptoms of premenstrual syndrome.

Selenium

Selenium is a trace mineral with antioxidant properties, especially when combined with vitamin E. It also helps maintain the immune system.

Dietary sources of selenium include milk, poultry, fish, organ meats and whole-grain products. The amount of selenium in these foods varies greatly, dependent on amounts of the mineral in the soil.

Low selenium levels may contribute to atherosclerosis, hypothyroidism and certain cancers. Cigarette smoking and alcohol abuse both lower selenium levels.

Our take

The recommended dietary allowance of selenium is small — 55 micrograms (mcg) daily. If you take supplements, don't take more than 200 mcg a day. Selenium deficiency is rare and usually associated with severe gastrointestinal problems that affect absorption. Although preliminary test results look promising, don't take selenium in large doses to prevent cancer.

What the research says

Research suggests that selenium may help prevent cancer and, possibly, heart disease. A large study was launched to determine if selenium and vitamin E can help protect against prostate cancer, but results aren't due for several more years. There have also been preliminary studies on selenium with respect to asthma, arthritis, infertility and the prevention of infection.

Zinc

Zinc is a trace mineral found in almost every cell in the human body. It's essential for normal growth, development and sexual maturation, and helps regulate appetite, stress level, and sense of taste and smell. Zinc plays an essential role in the immune system and also has antioxidant properties.

Zinc must be obtained through diet because the body doesn't produce enough of it. Dietary sources include meat, fish, poultry, liver, milk, wheat germ, whole-grain products and fortified cereals. The recommended dietary allowance for adult males is 11 milligrams (mg) of zinc and for adult women 8 mg.

Supplements may be needed for severe deficiencies resulting from malnutrition, alcohol abuse, liver cirrhosis and certain digestive disorders.

Avoid long-term high doses of zinc, which can lower high-density lipoprotein (HDL or "good") cholesterol, suppress the immune system, and interfere with the absorption of copper, which may result in anemia.

Our take

Whether zinc can prevent or lessen a cold isn't clear. At this point, taking zinc tablets generally isn't recommended unless you have a severe deficiency. Vegetarians and some older adults may be able to correct mild zinc deficiencies with multivitamins containing zinc.

Zinc is important to your diet, but try to get the mineral through whole foods. Until more research becomes available, it's best not to exceed the recommended dietary allowance.

What the research says

Here's what some studies have found:

Common cold

Studies conflict on whether zinc lozenges reduce the duration and severity of cold symptoms. Some studies indicate that taking a daily multivitamin-mineral supplement may increase the immune response in older adults while other studies suggest this may weaken the immune response.

Healing

Zinc deficiency can slow the healing process. Studies show that zinc supplements can help heal skin ulcers and bed sores in people with low zinc levels, but the supplements don't appear as effective when zinc levels are normal.

Other

Preliminary results suggest that zinc may have some beneficial effects on sickle cell anemia, attention-deficit disorder, Down's syndrome and herpes simplex virus, but more research is needed.

Saving your eyesight

A large study called the Age-Related Eye Disease Study found that taking a combination of certain vitamins and minerals may slow the progression of age-related macular degeneration. Among people with macular degeneration who took a combination of vitamin C, vitamin E, beta carotene and zinc, advancement of the disease was reduced by up to 25 percent. Large doses were used in the study. Several commercial products are available that mimic the doses used in the study. Discuss with your doctor whether it makes sense for you to take one of these multi-ingredient preparations.

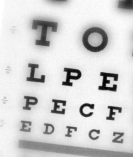

Hormones and other compounds

Coenzyme Q10

Coenzyme Q10 (CoQ10) is used to produce energy for cell development and maintenance. The compound also has strong antioxidant qualities.

CoQ10 is manufactured by the body, although it may be found in certain foods such as meat and fish.

This popular supplement is taken to treat disorders such as heart disease, high blood pressure, asthma, migraines, Parkinson's disease and certain cancers. It's also believed to help prevent aging and memory loss, and to improve exercise performance.

Our take

There's some intriguing — though preliminary — evidence that CoQ10 may be beneficial for treating conditions such as congestive heart failure, high blood pressure and Parkinson's disease. It also may help prevent statin-induced myopathy, a condition that can arise from use of statin cholesterol medications. Take the supplements under a doctor's supervision.

What the research says

Preliminary studies suggest that CoQ10 may improve symptoms of Parkinson's disease. Other studies examining the effect of CoQ10 on Alzheimer's disease, indicate generally positive results. Use of CoQ10 for treatment of cardiovascular conditions have produced mixed results. It may cause a slight decrease in blood pressure and it may improve symptoms of congestive heart failure. CoQ10 is also being studied as a treatment for migraines.

Dehydroepiandrosterone (DHEA)

DHEA is a steroid advertised as an anti-aging hormone. It's taken to build muscle, reduce body fat, improve sex drive and sharpen memory.

DHEA supplements are produced in a lab from an extract taken from Mexican wild yams.

The steroid was banned from stores in 1985, but legislation in 1994 permitted it back on the shelves as a supplement. Its use is banned by many sports organizations.

Our take

Studies suggest DHEA may be effective in treating mild depression, but there's little to support its claims of an anti-aging tonic. Long-term use and high levels may cause serious side effects.

What the research says

A two-year Mayo Clinic study published in 2006 found that DHEA has no effect on anti-aging indicators such as endurance, muscle mass, fat mass and insulin sensitivity, and no effect on quality of life. Clinical trials suggest DHEA may be useful for treating depression, but strictly under the guidance of a specialist. No studies have examined the effects of long-term use.

Dimethyl sulfoxide (DMSO)

Dimethyl sulfoxide (DMSO) is an industrial solvent, similar to turpentine, that's sold in some health food stores as a treatment for arthritis.

Some evidence suggests that DMSO can relieve pain and reduce swelling when rubbed on the skin. When used topically, DMSO may cause sedation, headache, dizziness, nausea, vomiting, diarrhea and skin problems.

Our take

DMSO may be no more effective than other topical, over-the-counter pain relief products for arthritis symptoms. Furthermore, industrial-strength DMSO — the kind generally sold in stores — isn't medical grade and may contain poisonous contaminants. For these reasons, arthritis experts generally don't recommend using this solvent as a treatment for arthritis.

What the research says

Nearly 40 years of medical research on DMSO has yielded conflicting results. The only use of DMSO approved by the Food and Drug Administration is for treating interstitial cystitis, a rare bladder inflammation. Some studies using animals found that joints treated with DMSO actually developed more inflammation than did untreated joints.

5-hydroxytryptophan (5-HTP)

5-HTP is an amino acid that the body converts into serotonin, a brain chemical that helps regulate sleep, appetite and mood.

Seed extract of *Griffonia simplicifolia*, a tree native to West Africa and Central Africa, is used to produce 5-HTP supplements.

5-HTP is used to treat a variety of conditions associated with low serotonin levels, including depression, anxiety and insomnia. The supplements are also taken for weight loss.

Our take

In recent years, 5-HTP has become a very popular over-the-counter treatment for depression. But any supplement that affects brain chemicals carries the risk of adverse effects. Use of 5-HTP isn't advised until more extensive study is undertaken. Individuals taking prescribed antidepressant medications or any other drug affecting serotonin levels should avoid 5-HTP completely.

What the research says

Research indicates that 5-HTP may have value in the treatment of cerebellar ataxia, a condition in which the brain is unable to regulate limb movements and body posture. Preliminary studies also support the use of 5-HTP in treating depression, fibromyalgia, headaches and obesity, but larger, well-designed trials are needed before recommendations can be made.

Glucosamine and chondroitin

Glucosamine and chondroitin are natural compounds found in cartilage — the tough tissue that cushions joints. They're used to treat osteoarthritis, a painful condition caused by the inflammation, breakdown and eventual loss of cartilage. Since the late 1990s, sales of these products have exploded, reaching nearly $1 billion a year.

Glucosamine supplements are made from the skeletons of shellfish (chitin). There are several forms of glucosamine. The form considered best suited for cartilage repair is glucosamine sulfate. Chondroitin supplements are made from cow and shark cartilage, as well as from other sources.

The two compounds are often administered in combination to treat osteoarthritis. (Sometimes, the trace element manganese is also included.) It's not clear whether this combination works better than either supplement would alone.

Our take

Glucosamine and chondroitin have become an extremely popular treatment for osteoarthritis. They appear to be safe and produce fewer adverse side effects than do medications such as NSAIDs. But how effective are they at treating arthritis? Many older studies gave very promising results. However, the results of a very large NIH-sponsored trial was mostly negative. The only individuals who appeared to receive some benefit were those with very severe symptoms.

While the studies may be conflicting, side effects from the supplements are few and far between. So far, no other treatments have shown promise in increasing cartilage. And it's still possible glucosamine and chondroitin may help. Therefore, they may be worth a try.

What the research says

Results of more than 30 studies have produced enough mixed results that researchers aren't able to conclude that glucosamine and chondroitin improve pain and function in people with osteoarthritis of the knee. Glucosamine, though, has shown benefits for osteoarthritis in other joints. In some instances, it appeared to reduce joint pain and tenderness as effectively as did conventional medications and slow progression of the disease. Whether people taking glucosamine and chondroitin for longer periods have less joint damage compared with those taking an inactive pill (placebo) is uncertain and requires further study.

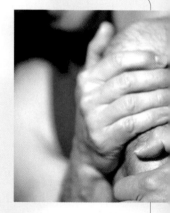

The National Institutes of Health (NIH) sponsored a four-year study in which glucosamine and chondroitin were used to treat people with osteoarthritis of the knee. Preliminary results of the study released in 2005 suggested that — when given separately or in combination — glucosamine and chondroitin generally weren't any more effective in treating pain than was a placebo. The study also found that a prescribed medication used for comparison was more effective than the placebo in relieving pain.

Meanwhile, a study conducted in Europe concluded that glucosamine was more effective than acetaminophen in reducing joint pain from osteoarthritis.

Glucosamine and chondroitin haven't been well studied for treatment of rheumatoid arthritis.

Human growth hormone

Growth hormone (GH) is produced by the pituitary gland in the central brain. Growth hormone stimulates and regulates childhood development, but levels of the hormone begin to decline around age 20.

Prescription medications, such as somatrem and somatropin, are available in injectable form. They're generally used for childhood conditions such as growth hormone deficiency.

Adults are using growth hormone supplements in hopes of slowing the aging process and keeping themselves young and energetic.

Our take

Growth hormone levels decline naturally as a part of normal aging. Although human growth hormone products may provide some physical benefits, their ability to slow the aging process is unclear. Many of these benefits could be better achieved through regular physical exercise, and at a lot less expense. On the Internet, many products are sold as growth hormone stimulants. None of their claims has been proved and the products should be avoided.

What the research says

Several small studies have shown that high doses of injected growth hormone can slightly reduce body fat and increase muscle mass and bone density. What's not certain is how these changes will effect overall strength, endurance and quality of life.

L-leucine

L-leucine is a branched-chain amino acid (BCAA), along with isoleucine and valine. BCAAs are used by athletes to increase endurance and energy levels during competition. BCAAs are also used to treat forms of encephalopathy, as well as anorexia in cancer patients.

BCAAs can be found in any dietary source of protein, such as meat, legumes and dairy products. Supplements, ranging anywhere from 5 to 20 grams, are available as capsules, tablets and powder.

Our take

Study results so far are mixed on the benefits of BCAA supplementation in athletic competition. It should be noted that BCAAs would only have positive effects for endurance athletes, not for athletes competing in events of shorter duration. Nevertheless, BCAAs do appear safe to use, with no serious adverse reactions reported.

What the research says

The idea behind BCAA supplements in athletics is that physical performance, particularly in endurance events such as marathons, is hampered by mental fatigue. Supplements such as L-leucine delay fatigue by blocking the manufacture of serotonin in the brain. Some studies indicate that BCAA supplements taken right before exercise are effective, while others show little or no effect.

Melatonin

Melatonin is a hormone that controls the body's circadian rhythm, an internal system that regulates when you fall asleep and when you wake up. It also helps control the release of female reproductive hormones, which determines the timing of menstrual cycles and menopause.

Supplements are synthesized from the amino acid tryptophan. The supplements are available as tablets, capsules, cream and lozenges.

Melatonin is used for a variety of medical conditions, most notably for disorders related to sleep, such as jet lag and insomnia. The hormone is a powerful antioxidant but at this point, no one knows exactly what it's capable of. Melatonin is advertised as a treatment for arthritis, stress, migraine, alcoholism, heart disease, cancer and symptoms of menopause.

Our take

Melatonin can promote sleep and appears to be safe for short-term use but its long-term effects are unknown. It's likely that your body produces enough melatonin for its general needs, and taking supplements regularly isn't needed. Melatonin may be used occasionally, such as to overcome jet lag, for people who have difficulty making sleep adjustments. Treat melatonin as you would any form of sleeping pill, and use it under your doctor's supervision.

What the research says

Here's what some studies have found:

Insomnia

Research on older adults suggests that taking melatonin at least a half-hour or more before bedtime will decrease the amount of time required to fall asleep. However, most of these studies have been short-term and not of the highest quality. Little is known of the long-term effects, or how melatonin compares with insomnia medications.

Jet lag

Studies indicate that melatonin, when taken on the day of travel and continued for several days, will help reduce the time required to re-establish a normal sleep pattern in a new location. Best effects seem to occur when traveling eastward, and when crossing more than four time zones. However, the symptoms of jet lag are variable and not always easy to assess.

Other

Melatonin has been studied as a treatment for cancer, headache, seasonal affective disorder and smoking cessation. Small studies have also examined sleep disorders associated with irregular work shifts, menopause, depression and schizophrenia. More research is needed.

Sleep enhancement

Several studies indicate that healthy individuals taking melatonin before bedtime will feel "sleepiness" and fall asleep faster. It's unknown whether it will help people stay asleep.

Omega-3 fatty acids

Omega-3 fatty acids are derived from food. They cannot be manufactured in the body.

Omega-3 fatty acids have been shown to improve cardiovascular health, helping to reduce the risk of heart attack, stroke, high triglycerides and atherosclerosis. They also appear to improve symptoms of rheumatoid arthritis — studies haven't found a similar benefit for symptoms of osteoarthritis. There's some evidence omega-3s may help improve cognitive function later in life and improve weight loss.

Dietary sources of omega-3 fatty acids are cold-water fish such as salmon, mackerel, herring, sardines and trout. Fish oil contains both docosahexaenoic acid (DHA) and eicosapentaenoic acid (EPA). Other sources of omega-3s are canola and soybean oil, flaxseed, walnuts and wheat germ.

Omega-3 fatty acid (fish oil) supplements come in liquid, capsule and pill form. Most people can take 3 grams (3,000 milligrams) a day without adverse effects. Taking more than this amount increases the risk of bleeding and may lower your immune system response.

Our take

Omega-3 fatty acids are essential for good health, but try to get them from your diet by eating fish. Omega-3 fatty acid (fish oil) supplements may be best suited for individuals with cardiovascular disease or an autoimmune disorder, such as rheumatoid arthritis. Fish oil supplements should be taken under a doctor's supervision.

What the research says

Here's what some studies have found:

Cardiovascular disease

Clinical trials of heart attack survivors found that daily omega-3 fatty acid supplements significantly reduced the risk of another heart attack, stroke or death. These benefits weren't so clear for people with no history of heart attack. A more recent study, however, found use of omega-3 fatty acid supplements provided no benefit to individuals with cardiovascular disease.

High blood pressure

Multiple studies report a small reduction in blood pressure in people who took fish oil supplements. This should be done under a doctor's supervision. Other approaches to lowering blood pressure, such as weight loss and salt reduction, may be more effective.

Lipids

There's strong evidence that omega-3 fatty acids can significantly reduce blood triglyceride levels. The benefits result from doses as low as 2 grams a day. Four grams a day provides even greater benefits. There also appears to be a slight improvement in high-density lipoprotein (HDL or "good") cholesterol, although an increase in levels of low-density lipoprotein (LDL or "bad") cholesterol was also observed.

Rheumatoid arthritis

Studies suggest fish oil supplements in combination with anti-inflammatory medications improve morning stiffness and joint tenderness for up to three months. More research is needed.

Probiotics

Probiotics refers to dietary supplements or foods that contain beneficial, or "good," bacteria normally found in the body. A common probiotic bacteria is *Lactobacillus acidophilus*.

These good bacteria compete with and inhibit harmful, disease-causing bacteria, helping to maintain a proper microorganic balance in your intestinal tract. Probiotic bacteria also help with digestion.

Most probiotics come from food sources such as yogurt and cheese, but they're also available as capsules, tablets, suppositories, powders and beverages.

Our take

There's growing interest in probiotics, spurred by their potential to treat various gastrointestinal disorders, but more research still needs to be done. In the meantime, there appears to be little harm in taking supplements, although a good, balanced diet should provide you with sufficient "good" bacteria. Probiotics may help ease symptoms of lactose intolerance.

What the research says

Probiotic supplements have been shown to ease side effects from treatment with antibiotics, for example, treating a *Helicobacter pylori* infection. Research has found probiotics helpful in managing irritable bowel syndrome, diarrhea and cirrhosis of the liver. Results of studies on use of probiotics for yeast infections is mixed. One study found that employees given probiotics missed less work due to illness than did employees not given probiotics.

S-adenosylmethionine (SAM-e)

SAM-e is a compound that occurs naturally in the human body. Among other functions, it helps produce and regulate hormones and maintain cell membranes.

SAM-e (sam-EE) isn't found in food. A synthetic version has become a popular, over-the-counter treatment for depression, arthritis and liver disease.

Our take

SAM-e has promise as an effective treatment for depression and osteoarthritis, but the long-term benefits and risks are still unknown. As with all supplements, it's best to consult your doctor before trying SAM-e. Two drawbacks are the inconsistent quality and high price of various products. Furthermore, SAM-e can interact with antidepressant medications you may be taking.

What the research says

Multiple trials indicate that SAM-e can relieve pain from osteoarthritis as effectively as nonsteroidal anti-inflammatory drugs (NSAIDs), with fewer side effects. It also appears to be effective for treating mild to moderate depression, although most of these studies were poorly designed. Only preliminary tests have been conducted regarding its effectiveness for liver disease, and no conclusions can be made at this time.

What makes a good study?

As you read through this publication, you'll find that quite often we say the product hasn't been "well studied," or it needs "more rigorous scientific study." So what constitutes a good study?

In general, the larger the study the better. When a study involves several hundred people or more — especially if the study lasts over several years — it gains more credibility.

How the study was performed also is key. Prospective double-blind studies that have been carefully controlled, randomized and published in peer-reviewed journals are the gold standard. What does that mean? Here's some information to help you out.

- **Clinical studies** are those that involve human beings — not animals. They're usually preceded by studies that demonstrate safety and effectiveness of the treatment in animals.

- In **randomized, controlled trials,** participants are usually divided into two groups. The first group receives the treatment being studied. The second is a control group. People in this group receive standard treatment, no treatment or an inactive substance called a placebo. Participants are assigned to these groups on a random basis. This helps to ensure that all of the groups will be similar.

- In **double-blind studies,** neither the researchers nor the participants know who is receiving the active treatment or who is receiving the placebo.

- **Prospective studies** are forward-looking. Researchers establish criteria for study participants to follow and then measure or describe the results. Information from these studies is usually more reliable than that of retrospective studies. **Retrospective studies** involve looking at past data, which leaves more room for errors in interpretation.

- **Peer-reviewed journals** only publish articles that have been reviewed by an independent panel of medical experts.

To date, many complementary and alternative treatments haven't been researched according to such standards. However, there's been a rapid increase in products and practices undergoing more rigorous scientific review.

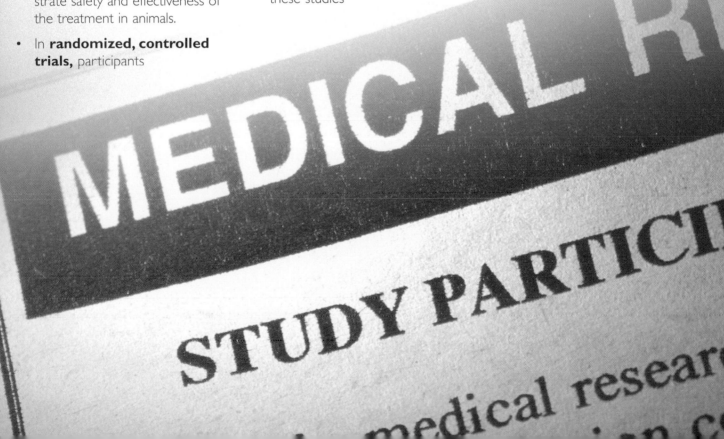

MEDICAL RE

STUDY PARTICI

medical resear

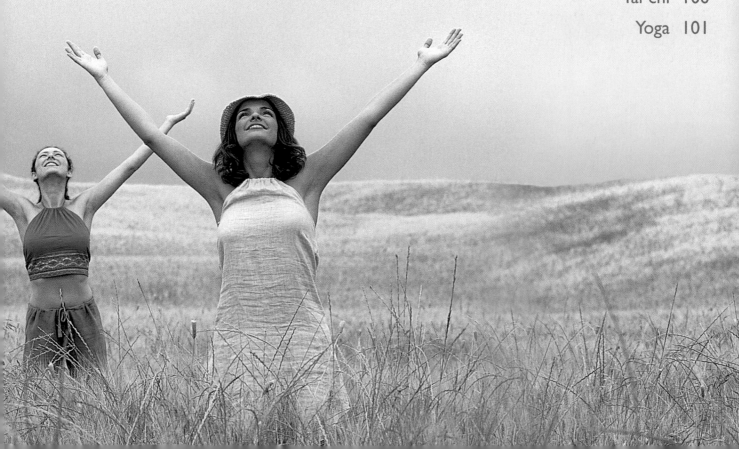

Chapter 4
Mind-Body Medicine

A visit with Dr. Amit Sood

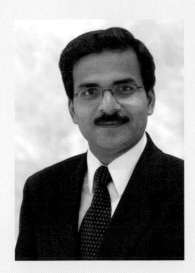

Amit Sood, M.D.
General Internal Medicine

"The power and speed of the mind is phenomenal. And there's no reason to believe that a mind that can sample the soil of a distant planet would not have the capacity to initiate processes to heal its own body."

A simple definition of mind-body medicine reads like this: "positively influencing the mind to improve the health of the individual." The belief that mind and body are intricately connected goes back centuries. But with the development of Western medicine during the 17th century, this basic "connected" approach to health and wellness fell by the wayside. As scientists explored the inner workings of the human body with increasing fascination, they discovered and introduced such fundamental concepts as germs as a source of disease, and medications (antibiotics) and surgical techniques as a way to treat disease — practices that remain central components of modern medicine. The study of human biology paved the way for great strides in medicine and continues to inspire innovative treatments. However, treating disease strictly on a biological level has its limitations, as reflected by the growing number of individuals turning to treatments outside of modern medicine.

Today, we're faced with several diseases, such as fibromyalgia and irritable bowel syndrome, that aren't curable with potent drugs or surgical procedures. This recognition — combined with increasing scientific study implicating the mind as one of several factors in the development of disease — has led to a resurgence of mind-body medicine and to increased interest in "holistic" health and healing.

The power and speed of the mind is phenomenal. And there's no reason to believe that a mind that can sample the soil of a distant planet would not have the capacity to initiate processes to heal its own body. An intriguing part of mind-body medicine — which is undergoing increasing study — is how mind and body respond to the healing effect of other minds. The positive benefits of interventions such as support groups may relate in part to the comfort and sense of security that comes with being part of a "tribe."

Mind-body practices have two core components. The first is to restore the mind to a state of peaceful neutrality. In this state, the mind achieves a state that's non-judgmental, efficient and adaptive to the needs of the individual. To reach this state, the mind has to shed negative experiences acquired over the years. The second component of mind-body medicine is to use this "ready" mind in a manner to achieve beneficial health effects. This might be through spiritual intervention (prayer), spoken intervention (transcendental meditation), or through practices involving breathing and posture (yoga) or soothing imagery (guided imagery).

As we learn newer and more refined mind-body techniques, it's important to recognize the simplicity of their underlying concepts. Interventions that at their core are based on the values of peace, forgiveness, sharing, selflessness, integrity and love help us achieve the outcomes we seek.

Biofeedback

Biofeedback is designed to help you use your mind to control your body. With the assistance of a variety of monitoring devices, including those that measure heart rate, skin temperature and brain activity, you can learn to control certain involuntary body responses, such as blood pressure, muscle tension and heart rate.

Biofeedback has been shown to be helpful in treating about 150 medical conditions. You can receive biofeedback training in physical therapy clinics, medical centers and hospitals. A typical biofeedback session lasts 30 to 60 minutes.

During a biofeedback session, a therapist places electrical sensors on different parts of your body. These sensors monitor your body's response to stress — for instance, your muscle contraction during a tension headache — and then feed the information back to you via sound and visual cues. With this feedback, you start to associate your body's response — in this case, headache pain — with certain physical sensations, such as your muscles tensing.

The next step is to learn how to invoke positive physical changes, such as relaxing those muscles, when your body is physically or mentally stressed. Your goal is to produce these responses on your own, outside the therapist's office and without the help of technology.

Our take

Biofeedback is, for the most part, widely used and accepted. It has the potential to improve symptoms associated with many medical conditions. It has relatively few risks and it's practiced in many medical centers. Provided you get proper instruction and supervision, biofeedback may be useful as part of a comprehensive treatment plan.

What the research says

Biofeedback is useful for treating many conditions. Studies indicate it has the potential to improve symptoms of asthma, Raynaud's disease, irritable bowel syndrome, nausea and vomiting associated with chemotherapy, incontinence, headache, anxiety, stress, high blood pressure and epilepsy. Research into its effectiveness in these and other areas is ongoing.

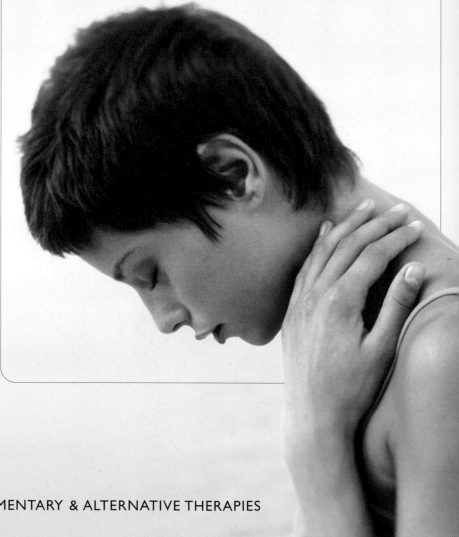

Guided imagery

Imagery is the thought process that invokes and uses the senses. You use it to see in your "mind's eye" a beautiful vista, or to conjure up aromas of your favorite foods. Guided imagery — sometimes referred to as visualization — has been used by cultures throughout the ages as a healing tool. It relies on memories, dreams, fantasies and visions to serve as a bridge between the mind and body.

Ancient Egyptians and Greeks, including Aristotle and Hippocrates, believed that images released spirits in the brain that aroused the heart and body. They also believed that a strong image of disease was enough to cause symptoms. Navajo Indians practice an elaborate form of imagery that encourages the individual to envision himself or herself as healthy.

Evidence of peoples' ability to use their imaginations to assist in curing their ailments was documented by both Sigmund Freud and Carl Jung.

Modern research has shown that mental images produce physiological, biochemical and immunological changes in the body that affect health. Researchers have found that imagery can change specific immune system responses that affect such things as white blood cell count. Imagery also has shown a potential to improve quality of life in some people with cancer.

Our take

Guided imagery gets a green light because it's an important tool in treating a variety of health problems. It provides benefits and it poses virtually no risk. Guided imagery is used in many medical settings to help manage an array of conditions and diseases from stress to pain to the side effects of cancer.

What the research says

Researchers using positron emission tomography (PET) scanning have found that the same parts of the brain are activated when people are imagining something as when they're actually experiencing it. For example, when someone imagines a serene image, the optic cortex is activated in the same way as when the person is actually seeing the beautiful vista. Vivid imagery sends messages from the cerebral cortex to the lower brain, including the limbic system, the emotional control center of the brain. From there the message is relayed to the endocrine and the autonomic nervous systems, which affect a wide range of bodily functions, including heart and respiration rates, and blood pressure.

Cancer care

Imagery has been used to reduce nausea, fatigue and hair loss, as well as create a sense of well-being among people with cancer.

Preparing for surgery

Research has shown that practicing guided imagery at least two to four times before surgery can reduce fear and anxiety and provide people with a greater sense of control. In a number of studies, individuals using imagery needed less pain medication and were discharged from the hospital one to two days earlier than were those who didn't use guided imagery.

Stress management

Imagery has been shown to be an effective tool for turning on the relaxation response in people who are feeling stressed, overwhelmed or physically uncomfortable.

How to do it

Guided imagery can offer relief from symptoms such as anxiety and stress simply by closing your eyes to the outside world. Imagery can empower the mind to create healing.

When first learning imagery techniques, many people find listening to a CD with guided imagery coaching to be helpful. Others choose to work one-on-one or in a small group with an individual who is experienced in imagery. After you've received a bit of training, you can perform imagery on your own.

Four steps are important in making guided imagery work for you.

Step 1: Relaxation

To create a desirable image, the mind must be cleared of all chatter and ego-based distractions. Loosen tightfitting clothing and find a comfortable, quiet place. Once you are quiet and comfortable, begin taking slow, deep breaths and releasing all random thoughts as you exhale.

Step 2: Concentration

Focus attention on your breathing as a means to clear your mind. If your mind wanders, acknowledge the thoughts, release them easily and effortlessly as you exhale. Then refocus your attention on your breathing.

Step 3: Visualization

Now combine a desired image with an intention and for the next several minutes, focus on this image. You may find that your mind wanders — this may happen frequently, especially during the early stages of visualization. When it does, bring your focus back by using a slow, deep breath.

Step 4: Affirmation

A positive affirmation coupled with the image will help to create a positive message that will be stored and easily recalled at a later time. Combining an image with a word or phrase may help to engage both sides of your brain.

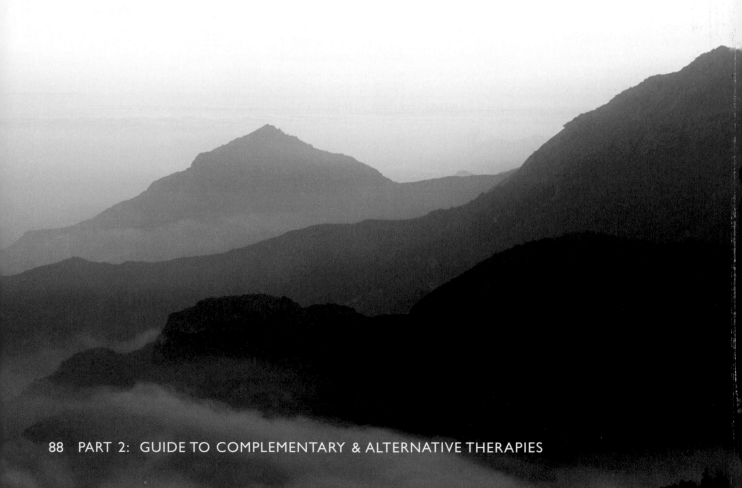

Hypnosis

Most of us have heard the term *mesmerize*. It comes from the name of an Austrian physician, Franz Anton Mesmer, who is considered the founder of modern Western hypnotherapy. Mesmer held that illness was caused by an imbalance of magnetic fluids in the body, and that this imbalance could be corrected by transferring the hypnotist's own magnetism to the individual.

The word *hypnosis* comes from the Greek word *hypnos,* which means "sleep." Forms of hypnosis, trance and altered states of consciousness have been used by many cultures and civilizations throughout history.

There are three stages or phases to the process of hypnotism. They are pre-suggestion, suggestion and post-suggestion. The goal during pre-suggestion is to open the unconscious mind to suggestion. During the second phase, a specific suggestion is presented to the subject, questions may be asked or memories reviewed. Finally, in the post-suggestion stage, after returning to a normal state of consciousness, behavior that was suggested during hypnosis may be practiced.

The mechanisms by which hypnosis works are not well understood. Changes in skin temperature, heart rate and immune response have been observed. Some scientists believe that hypnosis activates certain mind-body pathways in the nervous system.

Our take

While hypnotism is often portrayed humorously on TV and in films, it can be an effective treatment for some people. Research indicates that some individuals are more susceptible to hypnotism than are others. Some practitioners hold that the more open you are to being hypnotized, the more likely it is that you'll benefit from the therapy. Hypnotism may be a reasonable choice if you need help dealing with a chronic condition. Since it poses little risk of harmful side effects, it may be worth a try.

What the research says

Hypnosis may offer relief to those with pain associated with a number of disorders, including cancer. It is also used in treating a number of behavioral problems. In addition, it may be used to reduce anxiety before a medical or dental procedure.

Anxiety

Several studies show that hypnosis reduces anxiety. Particularly, hypnosis has been shown to lower anxiety before certain medical and dental procedures, with the effect lasting up to three years.

Behavior change

Hypnosis has been used with mixed success to treat conditions including insomnia, bed-wetting, smoking cessation and some phobias. More study is needed to determine the long-term effectiveness of treating these disorders with hypnosis.

Pain management

The National Institutes of Health has cited evidence that supports the effectiveness of hypnotherapy in the treatment of chronic pain associated with cancer, irritable bowel syndrome, temporal mandibular problems and some types of headaches.

Tension headache

Several studies have shown that some relief may be gained from the pain of tension headache with the use of hypnosis. However, comparisons with pain medication have not been done. Additional research is needed to establish whether hypnotherapy is effective in treating tension headache.

Meditation

The term *meditation* refers to a group of techniques, many of which have their roots in Eastern religious or spiritual traditions. Today, many people use meditation for health and wellness purposes.

In meditation, a person focuses attention on his or her breathing, or on repeating a word, phrase or sound in order to suspend the stream of thoughts that normally occupies the conscious mind. Meditation is believed to lead to a state of physical relaxation, mental calmness, alertness and psychological balance. Practicing meditation can change how a person relates to the flow of emotions and thoughts and may help you control how you respond to a challenging situation.

Meditation may be practiced on its own or as a part of another mind-body therapy, such as yoga or tai chi. Like other mind-body therapies, once you learn how to meditate, you can do it on your own.

Meditation may be used to treat a number of problems, including anxiety, pain, depression, stress and insomnia.

Our take

Meditation may be the perfect complement to the rush of a busy, complicated life. As the evidence supporting the use of meditation grows, adding it to your daily schedule may be just the antidote you need to deal with a hectic routine. In addition, if meditation helps to lower your blood pressure and reduce stress in your life, so much the better. The long-term benefits of meditation continue to undergo study.

What the research says

People practice meditation for a number of health problems. It's not fully understood what changes occur in the body during meditation, but the therapy is generally considered safe as long as it doesn't lead to delay in getting medical attention for an emerging or existing health problem.

Anxiety and stress

Various types of meditation have been used to treat anxiety. Studies have included people with chronic illnesses such as cancer. While benefits have been observed, conclusive evidence that meditation reduces anxiety over the long term isn't currently available.

Asthma

Preliminary research of the use of transcendental meditation in treating people with asthma has shown some positive results. However, the studies are not considered conclusive and more research is needed.

Fibromyalgia

Some improvement in symptoms has been reported by people with fibromyalgia who practiced mindfulness meditation (see page 91). Better research is needed before a more definite conclusion about its effectiveness can be made.

High blood pressure

Several studies have shown that a program of meditation effectively reduces blood pressure in people with hypertension.

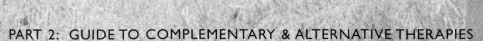

Different types of meditation

There are several different approaches to meditation. You may want to take a class to help you learn more about the various types and determine which approach is best for you.

Analytical meditation

The meditator tries to comprehend the deeper meaning of the object upon which he or she is focusing.

Breath meditation

This approach involves focusing on one's breathing. It's the conscious observing of every inhalation and exhalation, and the rising and falling of the chest. You may breathe in slowly through your nose and lightly purse your lips in order to feel the air flow out as you exhale through your mouth.

Mindfulness meditation

Mindfulness meditation has its roots in Buddhism. It's based on the concept of being mindful of — having an increased awareness and complete acceptance of — the present. During mindful meditation, you're taught to bring all your attention to the sensation of the flow of your breath in and out of your body. The goal is to focus on what's being experienced in the present, without reacting to it or making any judgments about it.

> **"** *The goal is to focus on what's being experienced in the present, without reacting to it or making any judgments about it.* **"**

This approach is used as a way of learning a more balanced response to the thoughts and emotions of daily life.

Transcendental meditation

Transcendental meditation (TM) teaches you to focus on a mantra — a sound, word or phrase — repeated over and over. You may repeat your mantra either aloud or silently to yourself. By doing so, you keep distracting thoughts out of your conscious thoughts. A goal of TM is to achieve a state of relaxed awareness or alertness. TM originated in the Vedic tradition in India.

Visualization

Visualization involves focusing on a specific place or object (see Guided imagery on page 87.)

Walking meditation

This form of meditation — called kinhin in the Zen tradition — focuses on the subtle movements used to stand and walk. You focus your attention on the soles of your feet, first as you stand, and then as you walk. Unlike sitting meditation, walking meditation requires that, for safety reasons, you pay more attention to what's going on around you.

How meditation affects the body

Practicing meditation has been shown to induce some changes in the body, such as in the body's fight-or-flight response. The system responsible for this response is the autonomic nervous system — sometimes called the involuntary nervous system. It regulates many body activities, including heartbeat, perspiration, breathing and digestion. The autonomic nervous system is divided into two parts:

The sympathetic nervous system helps mobilize the body into action. When you're under stress, it produces the fight-or-flight response. Heart rate and breathing increase, blood vessels narrow and muscles become tense.

The parasympathetic nervous system response is opposite to that of the sympathetic system. It creates what has been called the "rest and digest" response. The parasympathetic system prompts the heart to beat more slowly, the blood vessels to dilate, improving blood flow, and the digestive tract to increase activity.

Researchers studying the effects of meditation are focusing on the brain and how meditation may reduce the activity of the sympathetic nervous system and increase that of the parasympathetic system.

Getting ready

Most types of meditation require four elements.

A quiet place

Many people who meditate prefer a place with as few distractions as possible. This can be particularly helpful for those just starting to practice meditation. Those who have more experience may be able to meditate in places with more distractions.

A specific posture

Depending on the type of meditation being practiced, it can be done while sitting, standing, lying down, walking or in other positions.

Focused attention

Focusing your attention is an important part of meditating. For example, you may focus on a mantra — a specific word or set of words. You may also choose to focus on your breathing, or on an object such as a candle or an image.

An open attitude

Keeping an open attitude during meditation means letting distractions come and go without engaging them, without stopping to think about them. When distracting or wandering thoughts occur during meditation, they aren't suppressed. Rather, you gently bring your attention back to the focus.

In some types of meditation, the meditator learns to observe the rising and the falling of thoughts and emotions as they occur.

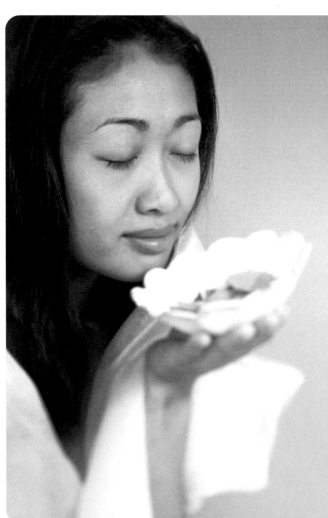

The soothing effects of aromatherapy

Aromatherapy, as its name implies, uses fragrant (essential) oils from a wide variety of plants in an attempt to alleviate pain, reduce stress, treat depression and promote a greater sense of well-being.

There are about 40 oils commonly used in aromatherapy. During an aromatherapy session at a spa, the oils may be smelled or applied to the skin during a massage. At home, you may add the oils to your bath water, burn aromatic candles or smell the oils while performing relaxation exercises.

Aromatic oils are usually mixed with a base, or carrier, such as vegetable oil, or they may be mixed with alcohol.

Several small scientific studies have found that lavender oil aromatherapy appears to have some effect in relieving anxiety. The scent of lavender is thought to have a calming effect on the nervous system. Lavender may also help some people bothered by insomnia fall asleep.

Aromatherapy has been studied in connection with improving quality of life for people with serious illnesses, but no firm evidence exists to its effectiveness in such cases.

Step-by-step instructions: How to meditate

One of the best ways to learn meditation is from an instructor, or you can try an instructional video or audio recording. You can also learn to meditate on your own. Here's an example of how to perform meditation at one of its most basic levels. It takes about 10 to 15 minutes. Try it and see how you do.

1. If you're able, turn on some soothing music and keep it at a low volume. Get comfortable in your chair or on the floor. Loosen any tight clothing. Let your arms rest loosely at your side. Allow yourself a few minutes to relax (pause).

2. If your thoughts wander, just let them while gently moving your attention back to the relaxation.

3. To begin, focus your eyes on a specific object in front of you, such as a tree, a picture or a candle flame. Notice its simplicity and its beauty.

4. Take time to notice your breathing, gradually slowing down the rate of inhaling and exhaling as you become more comfortable (pause).

5. Now relax and enjoy the feeling (pause).

6. Close your mouth and relax your shoulders, easing any tension that's built up (pause).

7. Inhale slowly and deeply through your nose. Let the air you breathe in push your stomach out.

8. Hold your breath as you slowly count to four. Then breathe out slowly through your mouth as you continue counting up to six.

9. Breathe in (three, four, five, six).

10. Hold (two, three, four).

11. Breathe out (three, four, five, six).

12. Breathe in (three, four, five, six).

13. Hold (two, three, four).

14. Breathe out (three, four, five, six).

15. Breathe in (three, four, five, six).

16. Hold (two, three, four).

17. Breathe out (three, four, five, six).

18. Breathe in (three, four, five, six).

19. Hold (two, three, four).

20. Breathe out (three, four, five, six).

21. Breathe in (three, four, five, six).

22. Hold (two, three, four).

23. Breathe out (three, four, five, six).

24. Continue breathing in (four, five, six).

25. Hold (two, three, four).

26. And out (three, four, five, six).

27. Remember, if stray thoughts enter your mind, gently return your attention to the relaxation (pause).

28. Now, as you breathe, silently and calmly repeat to yourself:

29. My breathing is smooth and rhythmic (pause).

30. My breathing is easy and calm (pause).

31. It feels very pleasant (pause).

32. Once you become familiar with how basic meditation works, you may want to close your eyes and focus on the music, or you can continue to look at the object you were concentrating on.

33. Continue to repeat to yourself:

34. My breathing is smooth and rhythmic (pause).

35. My breathing is smooth and rhythmic (pause).

36. I am peaceful and calm.

37. I am peaceful and calm.

38. Continue to take deep, rhythmic breaths. Let the tension fade away each time you breathe out. Let the music soothe you (pause).

39. If you've closed your eyes, gently open them and gaze at the object in front of you (pause).

40. Return to your day — peaceful, more focused and relaxed.

Muscle relaxation

Progressive muscle relaxation is designed to reduce the tension in your muscles. Your goal may be to reduce anxiety and stress, which may be related to conditions such as panic disorder, high blood pressure and depression. Progressive muscle relaxation may also be used simply to improve concentration.

Our take

Muscle relaxation is easy to do. It can be done just about anywhere, and it offers a way to reduce stress and clear the mind within just a few minutes. It's a tool that you can use after a difficult meeting, or to unwind at the end of the day. You might decide to use muscle relaxation by itself, or to combine it with another mind-body approach, such as guided imagery or meditation, to get an even greater effect. The great thing about mind-body medicine is that you can choose therapies that best fit your needs and style.

How to do it

First, find a quiet place where you'll be free from interruption. Loosen tight clothing and remove your glasses or contacts if you'd like. Progressive muscle relaxation is performed either seated or lying down.

Beginning with your feet and working up through your body to your head and neck, tense each muscle group for at least five seconds and then relax the muscles for up to 30 seconds. Repeat before moving to the next muscle group.

It's recommended that you perform progressive muscle relaxation at least once or twice each day to get the maximum benefit. Each session should last about 10 minutes.

What the research says

There's a growing body of evidence that supports the effectiveness of muscle relaxation in the treatment of some conditions.

Anxiety and stress

Various relaxation techniques, including progressive muscle relaxation, have been shown to reduce anxiety, work-related stress, and symptoms related to panic disorder. However, because studies tend to employ more than one relaxation technique and often have too few participants, more research on progressive muscle relaxation is needed to verify its effectiveness.

Headache

Some studies have shown promising results of relaxation techniques in reducing the symptoms of tension headache.

High blood pressure

In several clinical studies, relaxation techniques have been shown to lower blood pressure in people with hypertension.

Music therapy

While music has been used in healing rituals throughout human history, the modern, formal profession of music therapy was first recognized in the 1950s. It was during that time that musicians were called on to treat injured military personnel in the United States. Also during this time, various creative arts were used to treat psychiatric disorders.

Music can influence both physical and mental health. One aspect of music therapy involves listening to and then discussing a piece of music in order to help people express themselves. Music therapy may also be used in an individual setting to achieve a state of relaxation.

Music therapists are professionally trained and certified. They work in many settings, including hospitals, prisons, drug and alcohol treatment programs, long term care facilities and within hospices.

Our take

For many people, music occupies a central role in their lives. It revives their spirits, gets them moving and, in some cases, eases pain and suffering. Whether you listen to music simply for the joy and comfort that it brings, or you actively work with a trained music therapist as part of an overall treatment plan, music can be an important part of the healing process.

What the research says

There's scientific evidence that structured music therapy is effective in treating a number of conditions and disorders. Music therapy is sometimes combined with other approaches, including guided imagery, to achieve desired treatment goals.

Alzheimer's disease

Older adults with Alzheimer's disease and other memory disorders have been successfully treated with music therapy to reduce their aggressiveness and to improve their mood and willingness to cooperate in daily activities.

Autism

People with autism often show an increased interest in music, which may help in learning communication skills.

Depression

Evidence exists that music therapy can increase the effectiveness of some antidepressant medications.

Mood enhancement

Structured music therapy programs have been shown to improve mood in people facing burnout in their jobs and in people undergoing the rigors of cancer treatment.

Relaxation and stress reduction

Music therapy has been shown to reduce heart rate, blood pressure and tension in a variety of study subjects, including heart bypass patients, individuals recovering from a heart attack, and in babies being treated for lung and breathing problems.

Pilates

With its recent surge in popularity, you might think that Pilates is a hot new exercise fad. In fact, Pilates is a low-impact fitness technique developed in the 1920s by Joseph Pilates.

Designed specifically to strengthen the body's core muscles by developing pelvic stability and abdominal control, Pilates exercises also help improve flexibility, joint mobility and strength. They can help you develop long, strong muscles, maintain a strong back and improve your posture.

Many Pilates exercises are done with special machines. The earliest Pilates machine, called the Reformer, was a wooden contraption outfitted with cables, pulleys, springs and sliding boards. Using their own body weight as resistance, exercisers used the Reformer to perform a series of progressive range-of-motion exercises that worked the muscles of the abdomen, back, upper legs and buttocks.

Although machines are still used, many Pilates programs offer floor-work classes as well, designed to stabilize and strengthen the core back and abdominal muscles.

Instead of emphasizing quantity, Pilates focuses on quality, meaning that exercisers do very few, but extremely precise, repetitions. Exercises can be adapted according to a person's own flexibility and strength abilities.

Our take

While Pilates is a proven method of enhancing and maintaining physical fitness, very little research has been done into the effectiveness of Pilates in reducing disease symptoms.

Getting proper instruction from a qualified Pilates teacher may cost more than some other mind-body therapies. However, doing so can increase the chances that you'll get the benefits that you desire and that your Pilates workouts will achieve the desired effect.

What the research says

Research shows that when practiced regularly, Pilates can increase strength. It can also help to lengthen muscles and increase their flexibility.

Obesity and low back pain

Very preliminary research suggests that practicing Pilates regularly may help with weight loss when included in a well-planned weight-loss program. Pilates may also help reduce low back pain.

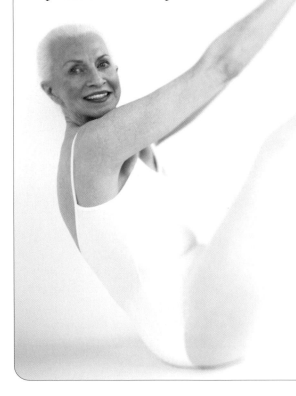

Relaxed breathing

Have you ever noticed how you breathe when you're stressed? Stress typically causes rapid, shallow breathing. This kind of breathing sustains other aspects of the stress response, such as rapid heart rate and perspiration.

If you can get control of your breathing, the spiraling effects of acute stress may automatically become less intense. Relaxed breathing, also called diaphragmatic breathing, can help you do that.

How to do it

Practice this basic technique twice a day, every day, and whenever you feel tense. Follow these steps:

- **Inhale.** With your mouth closed and your shoulders relaxed, inhale as slowly and deeply as you can to the count of six. When you breathe in, your abdomen should expand. Allow the air to fill your diaphragm.

- **Hold.** Keep the air in your lungs as you slowly count to four.

- **Exhale.** Release the air through your mouth as you slowly count to six.

- **Repeat.** Complete the inhale-hold-exhale cycle three to five times.

Our take

As with other relaxation techniques, relaxed breathing is easy to do, it can be done just about anywhere, and it's an easy way to reduce stress and anxiety without any expense.

Relaxed breathing can be learned through formal instruction, or you can follow the simple instructions on this page to get started. As with other mind-body therapies, relaxed breathing may be combined with guided imagery or meditation. There's little risk in giving it a try.

What the research says

There's evidence that relaxed breathing can help in the treatment of some diseases and conditions.

Angina

Preliminary research in people with angina suggests that some relaxation techniques may help reduce the frequency of angina attacks, reducing the need for medication. Additional studies are needed to confirm these findings.

Anxiety and stress

Relaxation techniques including relaxed breathing have been shown to help reduce anxiety and stress in people with panic disorder, work-related stress and some phobias.

High blood pressure

Relaxation techniques, such as relaxed breathing, may be combined with conventional therapy to reduce blood pressure and heart rate in people with high blood pressure.

Nausea and vomiting

Early research suggests that relaxation techniques may help reduce nausea and vomiting related to cancer chemotherapy.

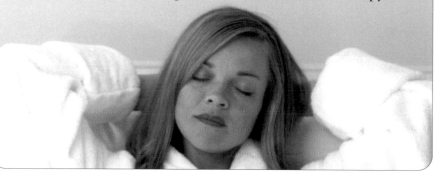

Spirituality and prayer

Spirituality has many definitions, but at its core it helps to give our lives context. Spirituality isn't necessarily connected to a specific belief system or even religious worship. Instead, it arises from your connection with yourself and with others, the development of your personal value system, and your search for meaning in life.

For many, this takes the form of religious observance, prayer, meditation or a belief in a higher power. For others, it can be found in nature, music, art or a secular community. Spirituality is different for everyone.

Spirituality begins with your relationship with yourself, is nurtured by your relationships with others, and culminates in a sense of purpose in life.

Realizing this, two of the best ways to cultivate your spirituality are to improve your self-esteem and to foster relationships with those important to you. This can lead to a deepened sense of your place in life and in the greater good.

Many people use prayer for their own health concerns and for those of others. In many religious institutions, prayer groups pray for members of their community who are sick.

Scientific investigation of the effectiveness of prayer in health settings has just begun. Evidence to date is inconclusive. However, there is some reason to believe that religious affiliation and practices are associated with better health and longer life.

Our take

We are complex beings with mind, body and spirit intertwined. For many of us, our busy lives mean that spirituality sometimes gets neglected until we're confronted by a major illness. But it doesn't matter so much what brings us back to our spirituality. It's just important that we nurture all aspects of our being in our quest to stay healthy. Find ways to energize your spirit, as well as your mind and body. Doing so can bring a healthy balance to your life.

What the research says

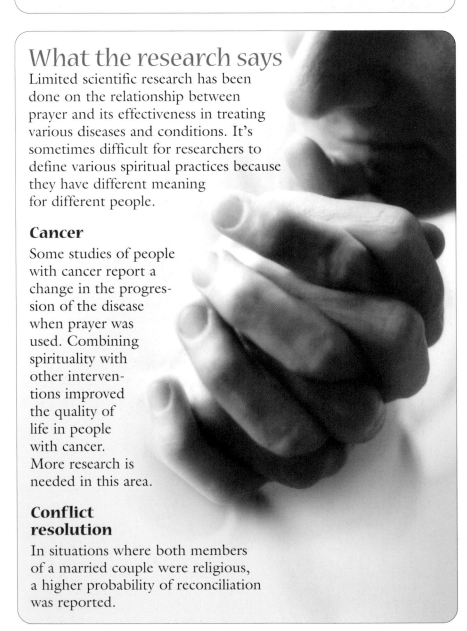

Limited scientific research has been done on the relationship between prayer and its effectiveness in treating various diseases and conditions. It's sometimes difficult for researchers to define various spiritual practices because they have different meaning for different people.

Cancer

Some studies of people with cancer report a change in the progression of the disease when prayer was used. Combining spirituality with other interventions improved the quality of life in people with cancer. More research is needed in this area.

Conflict resolution

In situations where both members of a married couple were religious, a higher probability of reconciliation was reported.

Spirituality: What's in it for you?

You may get many benefits from incorporating spirituality into your life. Spirituality can help you:

Focus on personal goals. Cultivating your spirituality may help uncover what's most meaningful in your life. By clarifying what's important, you can eliminate stress by focusing less on unimportant things that can sometimes consume you.

Connect to the world. The more you feel you have a purpose in the world, the less solitary you feel — even when you're alone. This can lead to an inner peace during difficult times.

Release control. When you feel part of a greater whole, you realize that you aren't responsible for everything that happens in life. You can share the burden of tough times as well as the joys of life's blessings with those around you.

Expand your support network. Whether you find spirituality in a church, mosque or synagogue, in your family, or in walks with a friend, this sharing of spiritual expression can help build strong relationships.

Lead a healthier life. Some research appears to indicate that people who consider themselves spiritual are often better able to cope with daily stress and to heal from illness or addiction.

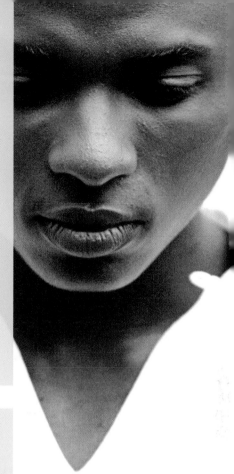

Becoming more spiritual

If you want to strengthen your spirituality but aren't sure how to do it, here are some suggestions you might try:

- Practice prayer, meditation and relaxation techniques to access your inner wisdom and help you focus your thoughts.

- Keep a journal to help you express your feelings and record your progress.

- Seek out a trusted adviser or friend — preferably someone who has had similar life experiences — who can help you discover what's important to you in life.

- Read inspirational stories or essays to help you evaluate different philosophies of life.

- Talk to others whose spiritual lives you admire. Ask questions to find out how they found their way to a fulfilling spiritual life.

- Be open to new experiences. If you are exploring organized religion, remember to consider a variety of different faith traditions. If your spirituality is more secular, you might consider expanding your horizons with new experiences in the arts.

> *Some research appears to indicate that people who consider themselves spiritual are often better able to cope with daily stress and to heal from illness or addiction.*

Nurturing relationships

Relationships provide many benefits. To expand your social network:

- Develop effective listening and communication skills.

- Make relationships with friends and family a priority, and stay in touch.

- Share your spiritual journey with loved ones.

- Seek out others with similar beliefs, and engage in conversation to learn from each other.

- Volunteer within your community.

- See the good in people and in yourself.

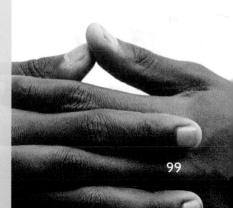

Tai chi

Tai chi (TIE-chee) is sometimes described as "meditation in motion." Originally developed in China as a form of self-defense, this graceful form of exercise has existed for about 2,000 years. It's becoming increasingly popular around the world, both as a basic exercise program and as a complement to other health care methods. Health benefits include stress reduction, greater balance and increased flexibility — especially for older adults.

To do tai chi, you perform a defined series of postures or movements in a slow, graceful manner. Each movement or posture flows into the next without pausing.

If you're trying to improve your general health, you may find tai chi helpful as part of your program. Tai chi is generally safe for people of all ages and levels of fitness. Studies show that for older adults tai chi can improve balance and reduce the risk of falls. Because the movements are low impact and put minimal stress on your muscles and joints, tai chi is appealing to many older adults. For these same reasons, if you have a condition such as arthritis or you're recovering from an injury, you may find it useful.

Tai chi appears to offer both physical and mental benefits no matter what your age. It's used to reduce stress, increase flexibility, improve muscle strength and definition, and increase energy, stamina and agility.

Our take

When learned correctly and practiced regularly, tai chi appears to be a very positive form of exercise. It's self-paced and noncompetitive. You don't need a large physical space or special clothing or equipment. You can do tai chi anytime, anyplace. It's easy to do in groups or by yourself. Because tai chi is slow and gentle, it has virtually no negative side effects. You could strain yourself when first learning, but with proper instruction, this shouldn't be a problem.

What the research says

Tai chi can reduce stress and increase balance and flexibility. Some studies suggest that practicing tai chi may be helpful in managing a number of conditions, including high blood pressure and depression.

Balance

Tai chi has been studied for its effect on improving balance and reducing risk of falling in older adults. Results of these studies aren't conclusive, and more research is needed.

Cardiovascular disease

There's some evidence to indicate that tai chi may play a role in lowering blood pressure and cholesterol levels. Additional studies are needed to confirm these findings.

Depression

Using tai chi in combination with other therapies may help treat depression and anxiety. While initial findings are encouraging, more research is needed.

Exercise

Tai chi has been shown to improve aerobic capacity.

Yoga

If stress is getting the best of you, you might want to try yoga. This series of postures — sometimes named for mammals, fish or reptiles — along with controlled breathing exercises, has become a popular means of stress reduction.

Though the practice of yoga has been around for thousands of years in India, its popularity in the United States has grown steadily only over the last 100 years or so. Today yoga classes teaching the art of breathing, meditation and posture are offered nearly everywhere from health clubs in big cities to community education classes in small towns.

Yoga is part of the Hindu religion and a way of life. The ultimate goal of yoga is to reach complete peacefulness in your body and mind. While traditional yoga philosophy requires that students adhere to this mission through behavior, diet and meditation, chances are you aren't looking for a complete change in lifestyle but rather increased flexibility, relaxation or stress relief.

Yoga offers a good means of relaxation and stress relief. Its quiet, precise movements focus your mind less on your busy day and more on the moment as you move your body through poses that require balance and concentration.

Our take

Yoga is rapidly gaining popularity in the United States. It's an excellent way to counteract stress, anxiety, and to relieve the hunched posture that can come from sitting for hours in front of a computer. Practicing yoga regularly can improve your flexibility and balance. It's one of those activities that you can do alone or with a group, and it doesn't require a big investment to get started. The risks of yoga are low, which is all the more reason for giving it a try.

What the research says

According to the National Institutes of Health, yoga can help reduce stress, slow breathing, lower blood pressure, alter brain waves and assist your heart to work more efficiently.

Anxiety

Several studies have shown that practicing yoga several times a week can reduce the stress of daily living.

Asthma

Researchers have found that practicing yoga can reduce the need for medication in people with mild to moderate asthma.

Back pain

Yoga decreased symptoms of back pain in a well-designed study, with the improvement lasting for several months.

Carpal tunnel syndrome

In one study, people who used yoga and relaxation techniques in addition to wearing a splint experienced more relief from carpal tunnel pain than did people who used the splint alone.

High blood pressure

Several studies indicate that regular yoga practice can help lower blood pressure. However, it's unclear whether or not yoga is more effective than other forms of exercise for lowering blood pressure.

Osteoarthritis

A study of people with osteoarthritis of the hands who took yoga classes showed that they had less finger pain than did those who didn't take the classes.

Yoga cautions

Yoga, overall, is considered safe if you're generally healthy. Some yoga positions can put significant strain on your lower back and on your joints. See your doctor first if you have any joint problems or a history of low back or neck pain. You might want to avoid certain yoga positions depending on your condition.

Also see your doctor before you begin a yoga class if you have any of the following conditions, as complications can arise:

- High blood pressure that's difficult to control
- A risk of blood clots
- Eye conditions, including glaucoma
- Osteoporosis

If you're pregnant or nursing, yoga is considered generally safe. But avoid any poses that put pressure on your uterus, such as those that require you to twist at the waist. Some yoga classes are specifically tailored for pregnant women. Check with your obstetrician if you have any questions whether yoga is right for you and your baby.

Hatha yoga: A popular form of yoga

Hatha yoga focuses on physical poses and controlled breathing. Several versions of hatha yoga exist. The version you choose depends on your personal preferences. But all varieties of hatha yoga include two basic components — poses and breathing.

Poses

In a typical hatha yoga class, you may learn anywhere from 10 to 30 poses. More experienced yoga students might know many more, including more-advanced poses that require advanced stretching and twisting. Poses range from the seemingly easy, such as the corpse pose, which involves lying on the floor, completely relaxed, to the most difficult poses that take years of practice to master.

Remember that you don't have to do every pose your instructor demonstrates. If a pose is uncomfortable, or you can't hold it as long as the instructor requests, don't do it. Good instructors will understand. Spend time sitting quietly, breathing deeply until your instructor moves the class on to another pose that's more comfortable for you.

Breathing

Controlling your breathing is an important part of yoga. In yoga, breath signifies your vital energy. Yoga teaches that controlling your breathing can help you control your body and gain control of your mind.

You'll learn to control your breathing by paying attention to it. Your instructor may ask you to take deep, regular breaths as you concentrate on your breathing. Other techniques involve paying attention to your breath as it moves into your body and fills your lungs, or breathing through alternate nostrils.

Mind-body therapies and cancer treatment

Most people with cancer who use complementary and alternative medicine don't expect the treatments to cure their cancer. They may use complementary and alternative medicine to treat the pain associated with their cancer and control the side effects of treatment, such as nausea and weakness. Your doctor might recommend conventional medications or complementary and alternative medicine therapies, such as acupuncture or massage, for these signs and symptoms. These types of therapy aren't specific to cancer and can treat pain and side effects of many other conditions as well.

In general, these treatments aren't invasive, making them safer than other complementary and alternative medicine treatments. Still, talk to your doctor about these types of therapy before using them.

Acupuncture. In this treatment, tiny needles are inserted into your skin to stimulate your body's natural energy, or qi (pronounced "chee"). By restoring the natural flow of qi, acupuncture is supposed to help your body heal itself. Acupuncture is effective in treating pain and nausea in some people with cancer.

Aromatherapy. Proponents believe that fragrant oils from plants can affect your mood. About 40 oils are commonly used in aromatherapy. You can experience aromatherapy at home or at a spa, or apply oil during a massage. Though little proof of its benefit exists, aromatherapy is said to help pain, depression and stress, and promote a general sense of well-being.

Hypnosis. This relaxation method effectively relieves some chronic pain, and it may also reduce nausea and vomiting in people with cancer. Although you may look like you're asleep during hypnosis, you actually go into a state of deep concentration. While you're under hypnosis, your practitioner may suggest you focus on goals, such as controlling your pain and reducing your stress.

Massage therapy. During a massage, your practitioner kneads your skin, muscles and tendons in an effort to relieve muscle tension and stress and promote relaxation. Several massage methods exist. If you're currently receiving conventional chemotherapy, check with your doctor before undergoing massage. If you have a low platelet count because of chemotherapy, deep massage can cause bleeding or bruising. Certain types of massage and spinal manipulation can also be unsafe if the bones in your back or neck have been weakened by cancer.

Healing touch. Touch therapy practitioners claim to use their hands to transmit "energy forces" that can improve the energy flow that runs through you. By moving their hands back and forth across your body, practitioners claim to be able to locate and remove energy force disturbances. Practitioners believe this reduces pain and encourages relaxation.

Many other types of complementary and alternative medicine are promoted for pain relief. They include homeopathy, reflexology, relaxation, spirituality, and art and music therapy.

A note of caution: Giving up on conventional cancer treatment that has been proved repeatedly in clinical trials to help people with cancer can be risky and even deadly. Avoid alternative therapists who pressure you to forgo the treatment your doctor recommends for a treatment that's unproved. Your doctor can discuss with you the pros and cons of conventional therapy as well as which complementary and alternative therapies are safe to try for your particular situation.

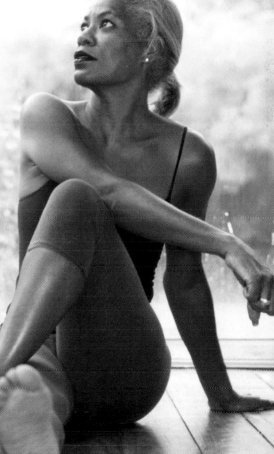

Chapter 5
Energy Therapies

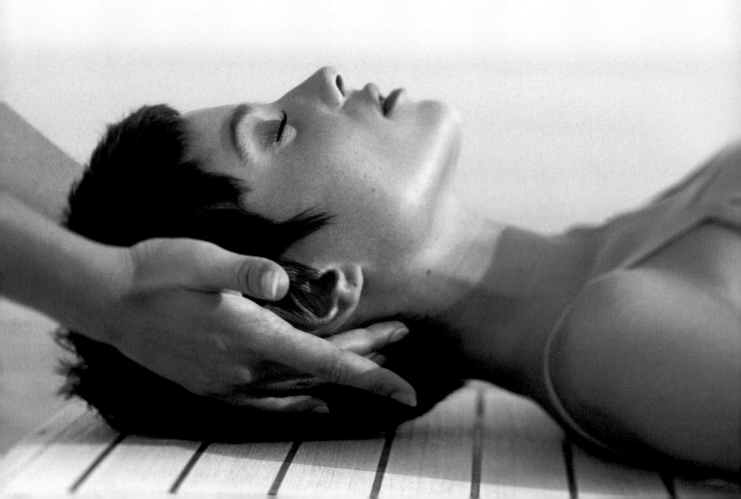

A visit with Judith Aufenthie

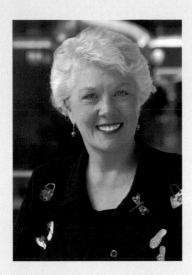

Judith Aufenthie, R.N.
Complementary and
Integrative Medicine
Program

" The goal of individuals who practice energy therapy is to help clear, balance and stimulate the human energy system, thereby promoting healing of the mind, body and spirit. "

Energy therapy is a fascinating form of complementary and alternative medicine that uses natural energy fields to promote health and healing. It encompasses a variety of practices such as acupuncture, healing touch, magnetic therapy and reiki.

Energy-based practices are founded on the belief that there are two types of energy fields: veritable, which can be measured, and putative, which can't be. Veritable energies use mechanical vibrations (such as sound) and electromagnetic forces (such as visible light, magnetism, and laser beams) to treat illness. Putative energy therapies, on the other hand, are based on the idea that human beings are infused with a subtle form of energy — a "life energy" — that flows through the body and surrounds it. When an energy pathway becomes blocked or disturbed, illness results. To heal the body, free flow of energy needs to be restored.

This vital life energy is known by different names in different cultures, such as "qi" in traditional Chinese medicine, "ki" in the Japanese kampo system, and "prana" in ayurvedic medicine. Other names used to describe life energy include dosha, etheric energy, fohat, orgone, odic force, mana, and homeopathic resonance.

Acupuncture is perhaps the most well-known form of energy therapy. It originated in China more than 2,000 years ago, making it one of the oldest and most commonly used medical practices in the world. Acupuncture is also one of the most studied forms of complementary and alternative medicine.

Acupuncture represents a number of procedures that involve stimulating an anatomical point on the body to ward off illness and promote health. This may be done by means of a variety of techniques. The technique most often offered in the United States is one where the skin is penetrated by a thin, solid, metallic needle that's manipulated by the hands of the practitioner. As the needle is inserted, the person receiving acupuncture may feel energized, due to activation of the body's life force energy, or relaxed, as the barrier interrupting the free flow of energy is cleared.

The goal of individuals who practice energy therapy is to help clear, balance and stimulate the human energy system, thereby promoting healing of the mind, body and spirit. When the body's energy system is in balance, it produces "wholeness" — physical, emotional, mental and spiritual well-being.

In light of accumulating evidence supporting the use of energy therapy for certain forms of healing, practices such as acupuncture and healing touch are gradually being integrated as part of patient care in some medical centers across the United States.

Acupuncture

Acupuncture involves the insertion of very thin needles to various depths at strategic points on your body. Acupuncture originated in China thousands of years ago, but over the past two decades its popularity has grown significantly within the United States. Although scientists don't fully understand how or why acupuncture works, some studies indicate that it may provide a number of health benefits — from reducing pain to helping manage chemotherapy-induced nausea.

Acupuncture seems to be useful as a stand-alone treatment for some conditions, but it's also increasingly being used in conjunction with conventional medical treatments. For example, doctors may combine acupuncture with medication to control pain during and after surgery.

Numerous past studies of acupuncture have been proved inadequate because of the difficulty of conducting valid scientific studies. Therefore, it's difficult to create a definitive list of the conditions for which acupuncture might be helpful. However, preliminary studies indicate that acupuncture may help relieve symptoms associated with a variety of diseases and conditions, including low back pain, headaches, migraines, osteoarthritis and fibromyalgia.

Our take

Acupuncture has been used at Mayo Clinic since the 1970s in a variety of treatment settings. Mayo Clinic also has a licensed acupuncturist on staff. When performed properly by trained practitioners, acupuncture has proved to be an effective therapy. In 1997, the National Institutes of Health recognized that acupuncture was being practiced widely throughout the United States and identified several conditions for which it may be recommended.

What the research says

Research shows that acupuncture is effective in treating a number of medical problems.

Fibromyalgia

In a 2006 Mayo Clinic study, acupuncture significantly improved symptoms of fibromyalgia.

Nausea and vomiting

Acupuncture can help reduce nausea and vomiting in people who are receiving chemotherapy. It may also help reduce nausea and vomiting from other causes, including pregnancy.

Osteoarthritis

Acupuncture has shown mixed benefits when used to treat osteoarthritis of the knee, hip and back. Some studies suggest it may provide considerable pain relief, while other studies show no benefit. One recent study of people with osteoarthritis of the knee showed a 40 percent decrease in knee pain among those receiving acupuncture. There was also a 40 percent improvement in knee function in the acupuncture group.

Pain management

A number of studies have shown that acupuncture is effective in treating postoperative dental pain, pain related to endoscopic procedures, low back pain related to pregnancy and some forms of chronic pain, including fibromyalgia pain. Acupuncture has also been effective in reducing pain related to tennis elbow.

Smoking cessation

Results are inconsistent. Acupuncture isn't a reliable treatment for quitting smoking, but it may reduce withdrawal symptoms.

How does acupuncture work?

Traditional Chinese medicine is based on the belief that the body contains a vital life energy, called qi (chee), which runs along pathways within the body. Imbalances in the flow of qi are thought to cause illness.

These life-energy pathways are called meridians and are accessible at approximately 400 different locations, or points, on the body.

Practitioners of acupuncture attempt to rebalance your energy flow by inserting extremely fine needles into these points in various combinations. This allows your body's natural healing mechanisms to take over.

A typical session

Acupuncture therapy usually involves a series of weekly or biweekly treatments in an outpatient setting. It's common to have up to 12 treatments in total.

Each visit typically includes an exam, an assessment of your current condition, insertion of the needles and a discussion of self-care tips. A typical visit usually lasts 30 to 60 minutes.

During a session, the practitioner should use sterilized, individually wrapped stainless steel needles that are used only once and then thrown away. You may feel a brief, sharp sensation when the needle is inserted, but generally the procedure isn't painful.

It's common to feel a deep aching sensation when the needle reaches the correct spot. After placement, the needles are sometimes gently moved or stimulated with electricity or heat.

Some people are energized by the treatment, while it makes others feel relaxed.

Inside the body

According to the National Institutes of Health, researchers are studying at least three possible explanations for how acupuncture may work:

- **Opioid release.** During acupuncture, endorphins that are part of your body's natural pain-control system may be released into your central nervous system — your brain and spinal cord. This reduces pain much like taking a pain medication.

- **Spinal cord stimulation.** Acupuncture may stimulate the nerves in your spinal cord to release pain-suppressing neurotransmitters. This has sometimes been called the "gate theory."

During a session, the practitioner should use sterilized, individually wrapped stainless steel needles that are used only once and then thrown away.

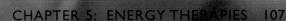

- **Blood flow changes.** Acupuncture needles may increase the amount of blood flow in the area around the needle. The increased blood flow may supply additional nutrients or remove toxic substances, or both, promoting healing.

Pros and cons

As with most medical therapies, acupuncture has benefits and risks. It's safe when performed properly, and it has few side effects. It can be useful as a complement to other treatments. It may also be an alter-

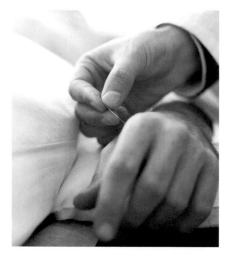

native to controlling pain if you don't respond to or don't want to take pain medications.

Acupuncture isn't safe if you have a bleeding disorder or if you're taking blood thinners. The most common side effects

of acupuncture are soreness, bleeding or bruising at the needle sites. Rarely, a needle may break or an internal organ might be injured. If needles are reused, infectious diseases may be accidentally transmitted. However, these risks are low in the hands of a competent, certified acupuncture practitioner.

Cost

Acupuncture is a form of complementary and alternative medicine that is sometimes covered by insurance.

However, you should check with your insurance company before you begin treatment to see whether acupuncture will be covered for your condition. Some insurance companies require preauthorization for acupuncture.

Choosing an acupuncture practitioner

In the United States, acupuncture services are offered by two types of medical professionals:

- **Medical doctors.** About 3,000 medical doctors use acupuncture as part of their clinical practice. Most states require that these doctors have 200 to 300 hours of acupuncture training in addition to their medical training.

- **Certified acupuncturists.** About 11,000 certified acupuncturists who aren't medical doctors practice acupuncture in the United States. To be fully certified, these professionals complete between 2,000 and 3,000 hours of training in one of several independently accredited master's degree programs. They also must successfully complete board exams conducted by a national acupuncture accreditation agency, the National Certification Commission for Acupuncture and Oriental Medicine (NCCAOM).

If you're considering acupuncture, do the same things you would do if you were choosing a doctor:

- Ask people you trust for recommendations.

- Check the practitioner's training and credentials.

- Interview the practitioner. Ask what's involved in the treatment, how likely it is to help your condition and how much it will cost.

- Find out whether the expense is covered by your insurance.

Don't be afraid to tell your doctor you're considering acupuncture. He or she may be able to tell you about the success rate of using acupuncture for your condition or recommend an acupuncture practitioner for you to try.

Acupuncture and cancer therapy

Clinical studies have shown that acupuncture is effective in reducing pain in people with cancer. In one study, most of the people treated with acupuncture were able to stop taking medication for pain relief or take smaller doses.

However, because of the design and size of the studies, the findings aren't considered extremely reliable. Studies with stricter scientific controls are needed.

The strongest evidence as to the effectiveness of acupuncture is in the area of relieving nausea and vomiting associated with chemotherapy. In addition, several clinical trials are studying the effects of acupuncture on cancer and other symptoms caused by treatment, including weight loss, cough, chest pain, fever, anxiety, depression, night sweats, hot flashes, dry mouth, speech problems and swelling in the arms and legs. Studies have shown that, for many people, treatment with acupuncture either relieves symptoms or keeps them from getting worse.

Qi gong

The word *qi gong* is Chinese and combines the term *qi* (chee), which means life force or vital energy, and *gong* (kung), which means accomplishment or skill. Thus, qi gong can be interpreted to mean cultivating energy. It is used in healing and to maintain health. Qi gong is practiced widely in hospitals and clinics throughout China.

Qi gong combines gentle, rhythmic movements, breathing techniques and focused intentions. There are more than 3,000 styles of qi gong. The styles include tai chi and kung fu. Some styles are meant to increase energy, while others are used to cleanse and heal the body, or to emit qi to help heal others.

Studies conducted in China have shown extensive health benefits from the use of qi gong in treating conditions ranging from asthma to high blood pressure. However, these studies are largely anecdotal and not randomized controlled trials. No large clinical trials of the use of qi gong have been completed so far. As a result, it's effectiveness from a Western-medicine approach is still unclear.

Healing touch

Healing touch, also known as therapeutic touch, draws on ancient healing practices from a number of cultures, including Indian, Asian and American Indian. Healing touch may be combined with deeply held religious beliefs and practices.

During a healing touch session, the practitioner first moves his or her hands a few inches above the recipient's body. This is done to assess the recipient's energy condition. Then the practitioner gently touches the recipient in a way that's designed to move energy through the practitioner to the recipient, strengthening and reorienting the recipient's energy flow within and surrounding the body. The goal is to promote the body's self-healing processes by opening blocked or congested flow of energy.

Some people who have undergone healing touch have responded that the treatment resulted in having a more positive mood, lowered pain, reduced anxiety or an improved sense of well-being. A typical session lasts 20 to 30 minutes.

Proponents of healing touch claim that it's effective in treating stress-related problems, allergies, heart conditions, high blood pressure and chronic pain. So far, there's no hard data to confirm this.

Our take

We recognize that people perceive health benefits from healing touch. Some people find the therapy to be relaxing, and certainly relaxation is good for your health. However, beyond relaxation, there's limited scientific evidence that healing touch improves health. Because there's little risk in healing touch, whether to try the therapy is up to you, based on how closely it fits with your personal beliefs.

What the research says

Many small studies of healing touch have suggested it's effective in treating a variety of conditions. These include wound healing, osteoarthritis, migraine, and anxiety in burn patients. One recent review of 11 controlled studies on the effects of healing touch showed that participants in seven studies had positive outcomes, while those in three other studies showed no effect. In another study, the control group fared better than those who received healing touch therapy.

There is some impressive anecdotal evidence that health touch works. However, more study is needed to confirm these findings.

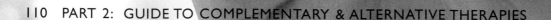

Magnetic therapy

Magnets have been used for centuries in an attempt to cure a number of disorders. During the Middle Ages, they were used to treat gout, arthritis, poisoning and baldness. In more recent times, magnets have been used to treat fibromyalgia, respiratory problems, high blood pressure and stress, among other conditions. By some estimates, people in the United States spend $500 million each year on various forms of magnet therapy.

There are numerous theories about how magnets might work to treat pain. One theory is that static magnets — made of solid metal — change how cells in the body function. Another is that magnets alter the balance between cell growth and cell death. And yet another is that because it contains iron, blood may be a conductor of magnetic energy. None of these theories has been proved correct.

However, in 1979 the Food and Drug Administration (FDA) did approve the use of electromagnetic therapy for treating some types of bone fractures. In addition, electromagnets have been studied for use in treating depression, knee pain from osteoarthritis, chronic pelvic pain, bone and muscle problems, and migraines.

The FDA still considers electromagnetic therapy as experimental for these and other uses.

Our take

Magnets are popular. Many people wear them thinking they can help reduce pain and other symptoms associated with conditions such as arthritis and fibromyalgia. Magnet therapy continues to be an area of active research. What's important to know is that there's a big difference between electromagnets and static magnets. Most of the current research involves electromagnets, which may hold some potential for treating conditions such as depression. Studies of static magnets — those used in bracelets, shoe inserts, mattress-pad covers, and so forth — have generally produced negative results, indicating no benefit.

What the research says

Research into the effectiveness of magnetic therapy is under way on a number of fronts. While this approach has shown promise, evidence as to its effectiveness is still evolving.

Arthritis

Several studies have looked at magnetic therapy applied to osteoarthritic areas or areas of degenerative joint disease to see if the therapy can reduce pain. Much of the research has focused on knee arthritis. Most studies have been small or not well-designed, and the effectiveness of magnetic therapy is unclear.

Bone fractures

Electromagnetic therapy has been used successfully for more than 25 years to treat bone fractures that don't heal well, called nonunion fractures.

Depression

Transcranial magnetic stimulation (TMS), being studied at Mayo Clinic, is used to treat people with depression who don't respond to more traditional therapies. Researchers hope to learn more about its potential benefits and risks (see page 112).

Fibromyalgia

A small Mayo Clinic study suggests TMS may be beneficial for treatment of pain associated with fibromyalgia.

Types of magnets

There are two types of magnets used in magnetic therapy.

Static magnets

Static — or permanent — magnets are the kind with which we're most familiar. They come in different shapes and sizes, but they all have a couple of things in common. They're made of iron, steel, rare earth elements, or alloys, and they produce energy called a magnetic field. This field attracts iron, and is strongest — and opposite — at each end of the magnet. Thus, each magnet has a north and south pole — a property known as polarity.

Unlike electromagnets, the strength of the magnetic field of a static magnet remains constant (static) and can't be varied.

Static magnets are the type most often marketed for health purposes. They're incorporated into shoe inserts, mattress pads, belts, bracelets and other jewelry, and head wear. The theory is that the magnetic field from a static magnet interacts in some way with your body to correct imbalances or reverse negative trends.

Electromagnets

Electromagnets consist of a metal core that's wrapped with a wire coil. When an electrical current flows through the coil, a magnetic field is induced in the core.

Pulsating electromagnetic therapy has been used for several decades to enhance healing of some types of bone fractures. More recently, researchers have begun to experiment with electromagnetic energy to see if it may help treat chronic pain, facial pain, headache, fibromyalgia and depression.

Biological effects

There's growing evidence that magnetic fields can affect various biological processes. Recent research has shown that some blood vessels that are normally dilated will constrict when exposed to a field from a static magnet, and that vessels that are normally constricted will dilate. This may lead to treating some kinds of tissue swelling and vessel blockages. However, there's no good evidence yet that magnetic therapy is effective in treating these conditions.

Treating depression with magnetic fields

Transcranial magnetic stimulation (TMS) is an experimental procedure that uses magnetic fields to alter brain activity. TMS is being used to help treat depression in people for whom standard therapies have not worked.

There are different ways to perform the procedure. But, in general, a large electromagnetic coil is held against the scalp near the forehead, often on the left side. An electric current creates a magnetic pulse, or field, that travels through the skull. The magnetic pulse causes small electrical currents in the brain. Those currents stimulate nerve cells in the region of the brain involved in mood regulation and depression.

You may feel a slight tapping or knocking sensation on your head during a TMS session. Although the procedure is generally painless, it may cause the muscles of your scalp or jaw to contract.

TMS doesn't involve surgery, and requires no anesthesia. You also don't need to be hospitalized. It can be done on an outpatient basis in a doctor's office or clinic that's doing a clinical trial for the procedure.

TMS is also being studied in the treatment of other conditions, including fibromyalgia.

Reiki

Reiki (RAY-kee) is made up of two Japanese words — *rei*, which means universal spirit, and *ki*, which means life force energy. As with other energy therapies, practitioners of reiki believe that disturbances in the body's energy systems can cause illness, and that by improving the flow and balance of energy, disease can be treated and health maintained.

In reiki, the practitioner delivers therapy through his or her hands with the goal of raising the amount of ki in and around the recipient.

During a session, the fully clothed recipient either sits or lies down. The practitioner's hands are placed either on or a few inches above the recipient's body. There are between 12 and 15 different reiki hand positions. Each position is held until the practitioner feels that the flow of energy has slowed or stopped, usually between two to five minutes. In addition to being delivered in person, reiki may be performed long-distance, with the recipient far away.

Recipients sometimes describe a deep sense of relaxation after a session. They also report sensations of warmth, tingling and sleepiness, and feelings of refreshment.

Reiki is used to treat stress, chronic pain, recovery from anesthesia, nausea from chemotherapy, as well as to enhance well-being.

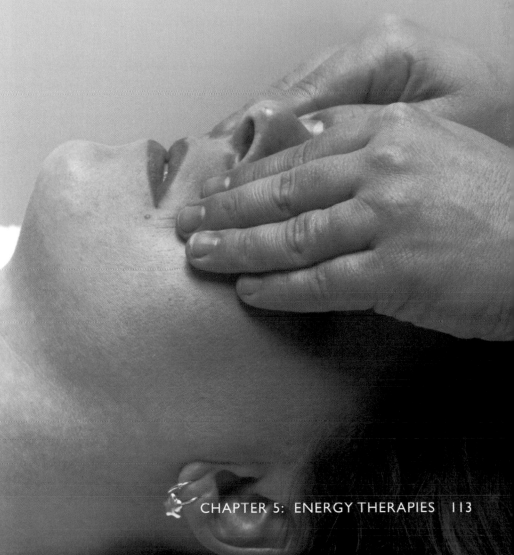

Our take

Similar to healing touch, the benefits associated with reiki may come from its ability to help promote relaxation. There's little, if any, health risk from the therapy. But there's also little evidence that it can effectively treat specific conditions. It's up to you if you think it's worth your money to give it a try.

What the research says

Reiki is touted for the treatment of many diseases and conditions. However, the practice hasn't been well researched and is lacking in scientific evidence. One study suggests that reiki may have some effect on blood pressure and heart and respiration rates.

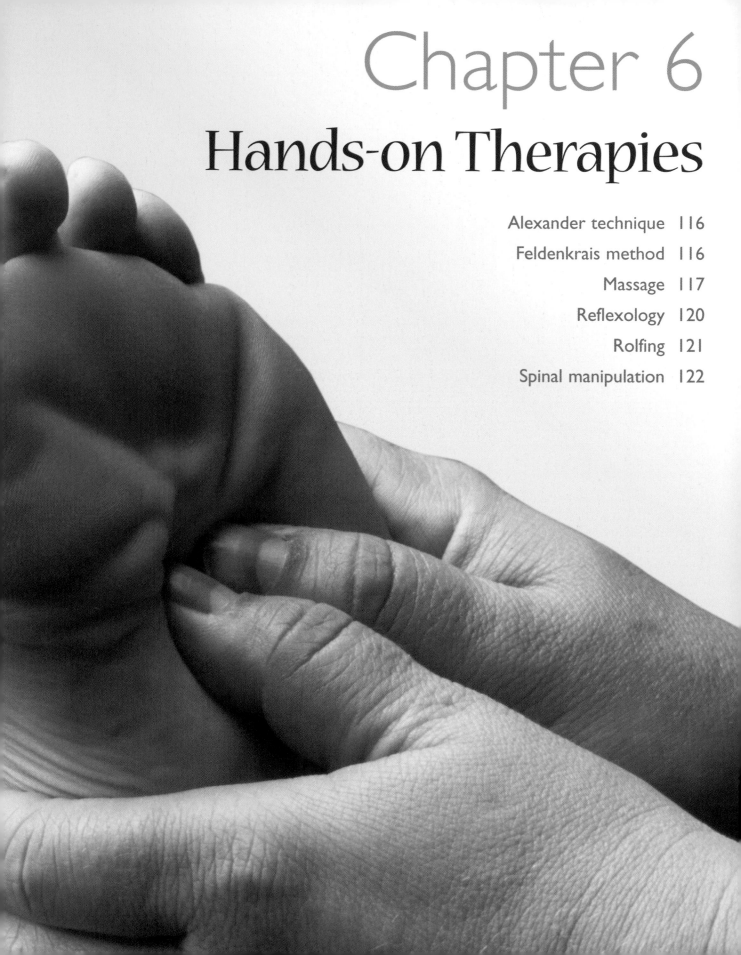

Chapter 6
Hands-on Therapies

A visit with Dr. Ralph Gay

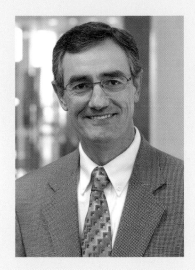

Ralph Gay, M.D., D.C.
Physical Medicine
and Rehabilitation

Surveys show that more than 7 percent of U.S. adults currently use chiropractic care and more than 5 percent seek massage therapy each year.

Hands-on therapies — practices such as massage and manipulation — have been used to relieve pain and illness for centuries. This group of treatments includes some of the most commonly used complementary therapies, used most often to treat musculoskeletal conditions such as back pain, neck pain, headache and arthritis. As a group, the providers of these therapies represent the largest contingency of organized complementary care practitioners in the United States and Canada, with the chiropractic profession alone having more than 60,000 members and performing approximately 95 percent of manipulative therapy in the United States.

Although once popular, hands-on therapies fell out of favor with the rapid growth of modern (Western) medicine during the last century. For years, the osteopathic and chiropractic professions in the United States struggled for acceptance, while in other parts of the world hands-on therapies became part of organized medicine. Gradually, these therapeutic tools experienced renewed growth in North America. Surveys show that more than 7 percent of U.S. adults currently use chiropractic care and more than 5 percent seek massage therapy each year.

Hands-on treatments — often called manual therapies — work by way of physical forces applied to the body. They have traditionally included massage, manipulation (joint movement caused by a thrusting procedure) and mobilization (joint movement without thrusting). As our understanding of the relationship between body structure and function has evolved, other therapies have been developed to help correct abnormal or inefficient motion. Movement therapies are thought to optimize the interplay between the nervous system and the musculoskeletal system and improve physical functioning. The Feldenkrais method and the Alexander technique are two examples of commonly used movement therapies.

Although not without risk, most hands-on treatments have limited potential for harm. When used appropriately, the most common side effect is local discomfort, which is generally short-lived. More serious complications can happen, though. Probably the most controversial treatment is cervical spine (neck) manipulation, which in rare instances can cause stroke (approximately one time in 1 million treatments). Fortunately, providers who use spinal manipulation — chiropractors, osteopaths and physical therapists — are some of the most highly educated complementary therapy practitioners.

The evidence supporting the use of hands-on therapies is variable. Some practices, such as spinal manipulation, have a large body of scientific evidence supporting their use for conditions such as low back pain. A few, like massage, are widely used but haven't been extensively studied. Yet others are less well known and are only beginning to undergo scientific scrutiny. Ongoing research is necessary to establish the appropriate place for hands-on therapies in today's health care system.

Alexander technique

The Alexander technique is named for F.M. Alexander, an Australian-English actor who believed in a link between posture, body movement and physical problems. Using the Alexander technique, you learn to become more aware of your posture and body movements. But unlike other approaches to movement, such as yoga or Pilates, the Alexander technique isn't a set of exercises. Instead, it's a way to heighten awareness of how you move, to improve your coordination and help you become a more intelligent exerciser. The Alexander technique is used to relieve pain, prevent injury and improve function.

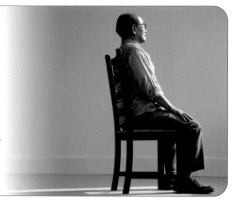

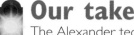 **Our take**

The Alexander technique is quite popular. Though there are limited data available as to its effectiveness, the risks are minimal. If you think it may help improve your coordination or relieve symptoms such as chronic pain, it's worth a try.

What the research says

Areas that have been studied include balance, chronic pain from the temporomandibular joint (TMJ), Parkinson's disease, and lung function in musicians who play wind instruments. Better designed studies are necessary to determine the effectiveness of the Alexander technique in treating these and other disorders.

Feldenkrais method

The Feldenkrais method uses gentle movements to develop increased flexibility and coordination. Though similar to yoga, the Feldenkrais method doesn't strive for correct positions, but instead aims for more dexterous, painless and efficient body movements. The goal is to create an awareness and quality of movement through body feedback rather than predefined postures. In group classes, which may be part of a physical or occupational therapy session, the instructor leads you through a sequence of movements — sitting in a chair, lying down or standing — that progress in range and complexity.

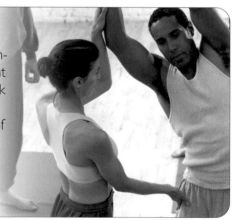

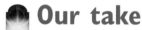 **Our take**

Similar to the Alexander technique, this form of movement therapy poses little risk. If you think it may help improve a musculoskeletal problem or symptoms of another condition, go ahead and give it a try. As to its effectiveness, there's not enough research to reach any definitive conclusions.

What the research says

The Feldenkrais method has been used to treat a variety of illnesses and disorders, including anxiety and depression, various musculoskeletal problems, and multiple sclerosis. In all cases, more research is needed to verify whether it's effective.

Massage

You might think of a massage as a luxury found in exotic spas and upscale health clubs. But did you know that massage, when combined with traditional medical treatments, is used to reduce stress and promote healing in people with certain health conditions?

During a massage, a therapist manipulates your body's soft tissues — your muscles, skin and tendons — using his or her fingertips, hands and fists. Massage can be performed by several types of health care professionals, such as a massage therapist, physical therapist or occupational therapist. Several versions of massage exist, and they're performed in a variety of settings.

A massage may make you feel relaxed, but it isn't likely to cure everything that ails you. And, if performed incorrectly, it could hurt you. Learning about massage before you try one can help ensure that the experience is safe and enjoyable (see "What to expect during a massage" on page 118).

Massage can relieve tension in your muscles, and most people use it for relaxation, relief of stress and anxiety, or to reduce muscle soreness. Massage can also cause your body to release natural painkillers, and it may boost your immune system.

Our take

Massage is a great complementary and alternative treatment. Almost everyone feels better after a massage. The treatment has been shown to help relieve pain and soreness and reduce anxiety. There are different types of massage. If you find one that works for you, you may be surprised at how quickly it can become a regular part of your weekly routine! While generally safe, there are some instances in which a massage may not be recommended (see page 119).

What the research says

Here's what some studies have found:

Anxiety

Massage reduced anxiety in depressed children and anorexic women. It also reduced anxiety and withdrawal symptoms in adults trying to quit smoking.

Cancer treatment

People with cancer who received regularly scheduled massage therapy during treatment reported less anxiety, pain and fatigue.

Children with diabetes

Children who were massaged every day by their parents were more likely to stick to their medication and diet regimens, which helped reduce their blood glucose levels.

Immune system

People with HIV who participated in massage studies showed an increased number of natural killer cells, which are thought to defend the body from viral and cancer cells.

Pain

Pain was decreased in studies of people with fibromyalgia, migraines and recent surgeries. Back pain also might be relieved by massage. However, back pain study results have been contradictory, and more research is required.

Sports-related soreness

Some athletes receive massages after exercise, especially to the muscles they use most in their sport or activity. A massage might help increase blood flow to your muscles and reduce soreness.

What to expect during a massage

No matter what kind of massage you choose, you should feel calm and relaxed during and after your massage. When you have a massage, expect to:

Answer a few questions. Your massage therapist will want to know what you want from your massage. Are you looking for help with a pulled muscle? Massage therapists will also want to know about any medical conditions you may have, so they can decide if massage is safe for you or how to make it safer.

Disrobe. You'll be asked to remove your clothes, or at least most of them. Your massage therapist should give you privacy while you take your clothes off and provide a robe or a towel to cover yourself. A good massage therapist will understand your modesty and keep you covered as much as possible throughout the massage.

If taking your clothes off doesn't sound relaxing or if you're pressed for time, try a chair massage. These massages are conducted while you sit in a special chair that slopes forward so the massage therapist can work on your back. It's often done in the open, rather than in a private room.

Be asked to lie down. Most massages will require you to lie on a padded table. Pillows or bolsters might be used to position you during the massage.

This allows you to relax completely during the massage. Music usually plays softly while you're massaged.

Have oils and lotions used on your skin. Some massage therapists use oils or lotions to reduce friction while massaging your body. If you're allergic to any ingredients commonly found in body oils and lotions, tell your massage therapist. You may opt not to use oils and lotions if you prefer.

Never feel significant pain. Pain that's more significant than just momentary discomfort could indicate that something is wrong. If a massage therapist is pushing too hard, tell him or her to lighten the pressure. Your massage therapist will expect feedback from you to understand how best to massage you. Occasionally you may have a sensitive spot in a muscle that feels like a

knot. It's likely to be uncomfortable while your massage therapist works it out. But if it becomes painful, speak up.

Spend about an hour. Most table massages last about an hour, though some may be shorter and others up to 90 minutes long. It's generally your preference.

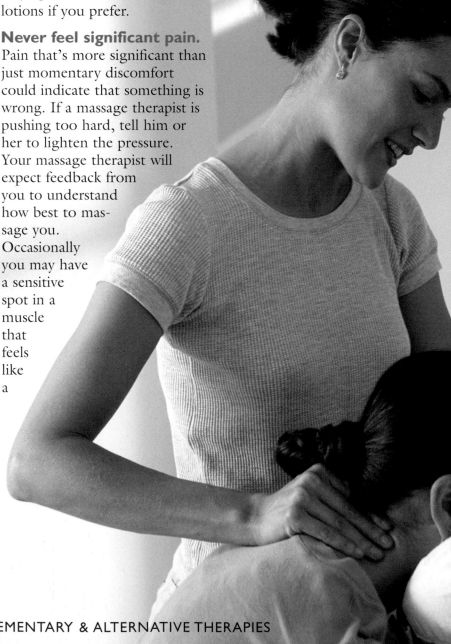

Chinese massage

Chinese massage, called tui na, is the oldest known system of massage. It's been used in China for 2,000 years, dating back to the Shang dynasty.

Unlike other forms of massage therapy, tui na is more closely related to acupuncture in its use of the meridian system. Through the application of massage and manipulation techniques at specific points on the body, tui na seeks to establish harmonious flow of the body's vital life energy — called "qi" — allowing the body to naturally heal itself. Qi is believed to run along an intricate system of channels, called meridians.

The term *tui na* translates into "push and pull" in Chinese. It's a series of maneuvers that include pressing, kneading and grasping, which range from light stroking to deep-tissue work. The maneuvers involve use of hand techniques to massage the body's soft tissues (muscles and tendons), acupressure techniques to affect the flow of qi, and manipulation techniques to realign the musculoskeletal system.

Unlike most other forms of massage, Chinese massage generally isn't a light, relaxing massage. It can be quite powerful and some people find portions of the massage to be a bit painful.

Tui na is generally used to treat injuries, joint and muscle problems, chronic pain and some internal disorders. It shouldn't be used for conditions such as a bone fracture or external wound or open sores. It's also not recommended for life-threatening conditions such as a cancerous tumor.

Avoiding potential risks

Massage is generally safe as long as it's done by a trained therapist. But massage isn't for everyone. And for some people it can even be dangerous. Discuss massage with your doctor before making an appointment if you're pregnant or if you have:

- Burns or open wounds on the area to be massaged

- Had a recent heart attack

- Cancer — you'll want to avoid direct pressure on the tumor area

- Deep vein thrombosis

- Unhealed fractures

- Rheumatoid arthritis in the area to be massaged

- Severe osteoporosis

Massage done properly rarely leads to severe injuries. Ask your massage therapist about his or her training and qualifications — some states require licensing. And if any part of your massage doesn't feel right or is painful, speak up right away. Most serious problems come from too much pressure during massage. In rare circumstances, massage can cause:

- Internal bleeding

- Nerve damage

- Temporary paralysis

Talk to your doctor and your massage therapist if you have any concerns about your risk of injury. Asking questions can help you feel more at ease.

Reflexology

The theory behind reflexology is that specific areas on the soles of your feet correspond to other parts of your body — such as your head or neck or your internal organs.

Reflexologists use foot charts to guide them as they massage, and then apply varying amounts of manual pressure to specific areas of the feet in an effort to influence a problem elsewhere in the body. Sometimes, reflexologists also use items such as rubber balls, rubber bands or sticks of wood to assist in their work. The practice was developed by William Fitzgerald, M.D., in the early 20th century.

Reflexology is practiced primarily as a form of treatment for a wide variety of problems. However, some reflexologists also claim to diagnose certain illnesses based on the condition of the soles of a person's feet.

Reflexology is sometimes combined with other hands-on therapies, and may be offered by chiropractors and physical therapists.

Our take

There's little risk involved in reflexology, and massaging the soles of your feet can feel good. But there's also not much evidence to indicate that the therapy can treat various diseases or symptoms, as its practitioners claim. Among most conventional doctors, the theory behind reflexology is a little difficult to grasp.

What the research says

Here's what some studies have found. All of the results require further research.

Anxiety

There is preliminary evidence that reflexology may be helpful in aiding in relaxation.

Headache

Some research has shown that reflexology treatments may relieve the pain of tension headache and migraine.

Premenstrual syndrome

Preliminary research has shown that weekly sessions for a period of two months reduced the severity of premenstrual syndrome.

Rolfing

Rolfing is a form of deep-tissue massage. It was developed by Ida Rolf, Ph.D., who called her work Structural Integration. It's based on the theory that the tissues surrounding your muscles become thickened and stiff as you get older. This affects your posture and how well you're able to move.

Rolfing practitioners use their fingers, knuckles, thumbs, elbows and knees to slowly manipulate muscles and the tissues surrounding muscles and joints in an effort to alter a person's posture and realign the body. The goal of Rolfing may be to relieve stress and anxiety, ease pain, improve posture and balance, or to create more-refined patterns of movement so that you can make more efficient use of your muscles.

Because it involves manipulation of tissues deep beneath the skin, people with bleeding disorders or who are taking blood thinners should avoid Rolfing. Those with broken bones, advanced osteoporosis, rheumatoid arthritis, abdominal disorders, and pregnant women should also avoid Rolfing. If you have any question about whether you might be at risk from Rolfing, talk with your doctor.

Our take

Some people find Rolfing to be very helpful, improving their posture or helping them to feel more limber. But the therapy can also be painful. If you have a specific underlying illness, such as advanced osteoporosis, the deep massage of Rolfing may also pose some risk. Therefore, it's best to talk to your doctor before embarking down the Rolfing path.

What the research says

Rolfing is used to treat many diseases and conditions. However, there is very limited research as to its effectiveness. It has been studied for the treatment of low back pain, cerebral palsy and chronic fatigue syndrome. The studies were small, and more reliable data are needed.

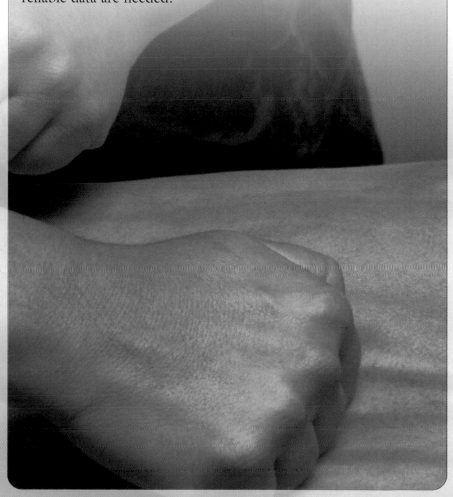

Spinal manipulation

Spinal manipulation is based on the premise that health and disease are directly related to the functioning of the body's neuromusculoskeletal system, and that with proper alignment of your bones, joints, muscles and associated nerves come health and healing.

Spinal manipulation — sometimes called spinal adjustment — is practiced by chiropractors, doctors of osteopathic medicine and physical therapists.

Spinal manipulation has been shown to be effective in treating certain musculoskeletal conditions, like low back pain. It's generally considered to be safe, but it's not appropriate for everyone.

- Don't seek spinal manipulation if you have osteoporosis or symptoms of nerve damage, such as numbness, tingling or loss of strength in a limb, hand or foot.
- If you have a history of spinal surgery, check with your surgeon before a treatment.
- Manipulation may be hazardous if you've had a stroke related to vascular disease of the arteries in your neck.
- If you have back pain accompanied by fever, chills, sweats or unintentional weight loss, see a medical doctor to rule out the possibility of an infection or tumor.

Our take

Studies have found spinal manipulation to be an effective treatment for uncomplicated low back pain, especially if the pain has been present less than four weeks. For this condition, spinal manipulation has become an accepted practice and no longer is considered alternative. Studies also suggest spinal manipulation may be effective for headache and other spine-related conditions, such as neck pain. There's no evidence, though, to support the belief that spinal manipulation can cure whatever ails you.

Select a practitioner who's willing to work with other members of your health care team.

What the research says

Spinal manipulation is an effective treatment for low back pain, especially shortly after the pain begins. After reviewing many studies, the Agency for Healthcare Research and Quality concluded that spinal manipulation may provide temporary relief from low back pain. However, the agency limited its conclusions to short-term treatment. There was little evidence long-term treatment was effective.

Spinal manipulation is also used to treat other conditions. There's some evidence it may improve headache symptoms or help relieve neck pain. As for treatment of nonmusculoskeletal conditions, such as asthma or ear infections, studies either haven't been conducted or haven't found spinal manipulation to be effective.

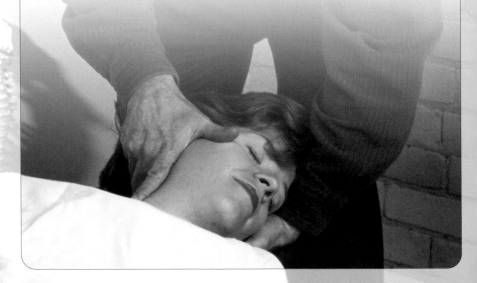

About chiropractic treatment

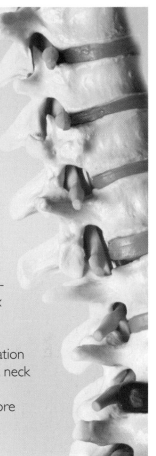

Chiropractic treatment is based on the concept that restricted movement in the spine may lead to pain and reduced function. Spinal adjustment (manipulation) is one form of therapy chiropractors use to treat restricted spinal mobility. The goal is to restore spinal movement and, as a result, improve function and decrease back pain.

During an adjustment, chiropractors use their hands to apply a controlled, sudden force to a joint. This maneuver often results in a cracking sound made by separation of the joint surfaces — not, as many people think, by "cracking joints." Although this sound is common, it doesn't have to occur for the treatment to be successful.

Chiropractors may also use massage and stretching to relax muscles that are shortened or in spasm. Many use additional treatments as well, such as exercise, ultrasound and electrical muscle stimulation.

As with any medical specialist, select a chiropractor who's willing to work with the other members of your health care team. Make sure you're comfortable with the recommendations, including how many sessions you'll need. For acute low back pain, four to six sessions are typically enough. Be questionable of chiropractors who ask to extend your treatment indefinitely.

When limited to the low back, chiropractic adjustment has few risks. However, manipulation of the neck has been associated with injury to the blood vessels supplying the brain. Rarely, neck manipulation may cause a stroke.

With increasing interest in complementary and integrative medicine, it's becoming more common to see chiropractors practicing alongside other medical providers.

About osteopathic treatment

Doctors of osteopathy are known as D.O.s, and you can find them in medical institutions throughout the country, including Mayo Clinic. Doctors of osteopathy are fully trained in conventional medical care as well as osteopathic medicine.

Osteopathic medicine focuses on the whole person — the mind as well as the body — rather than solely on a set of symptoms. It combines conventional medicine — including the use of prescription medications — with spinal manipulation and attention to proper posture and body positioning. Osteopaths use specialized manipulative techniques to facilitate the return of the body to normal motion and function in order to allow the body to heal itself. Osteopathic manipulation is usually more rhythmic and less abrupt than chiropractic techniques.

Osteopathic manipulation is designed to affect the whole person. Psychological changes are often observed after treatment, including changes in mood, altered nervous system activity and altered sensory experience. After an injury or illness, there's a natural tendency to focus on the part of the body that's injured or the origin of the illness, or to try to ignore it. Osteopathic manipulation attempts to put the individual back in touch with his or her entire body in order to aid in healing.

There's a growing body of research exploring the possible benefits of osteopathic treatment for a variety of health conditions.

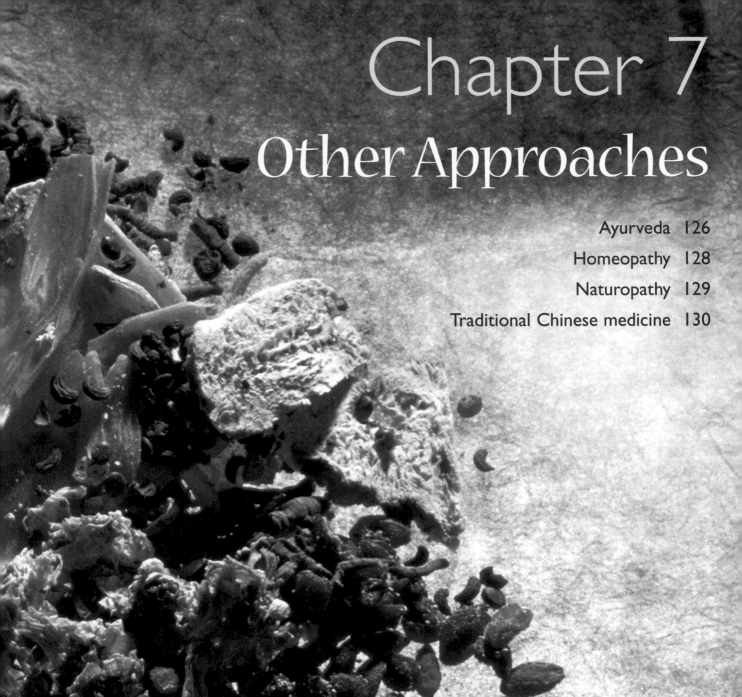

Chapter 7
Other Approaches

A visit with Dr. Ann Vincent

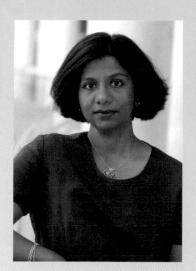

Ann Vincent, M.D.
Complementary and
Integrative Medicine Program

> *Common elements shared by most alternative medical systems are the beliefs that the mind and body are powerfully connected and that the body has the power to heal itself.*

In this chapter we discuss overall approaches to health and healing — complete medical systems — that are quite different from traditional Western medicine. The National Center for Complementary and Alternative Medicine refers to these practices as *whole medical systems*. Another common term is *alternative medical systems*. These forms of medicine are practiced by individual cultures and are largely based on traditional customs, many of which date back thousands of years.

Some alternative medical systems evolved in Western cultures, but most originated elsewhere. Examples of alternative medical systems that developed in Western cultures include homeopathic medicine and naturopathic medicine. Alternative medical systems that evolved in non-Western cultures include ayurveda, which originated in India, and traditional Chinese medicine. Other alternative medical approaches in use today include American Indian, African, Tibetan and South American systems.

Common elements shared by most alternative medical systems are the beliefs that the mind and body are powerfully connected and that the body has the power to heal itself. Treatments that comprise alternative medical systems generally focus on prevention and restoring natural "balance" to enable healing to occur. The systems have a strong focus on diet, exercise, sleep and daily routines — ayurvedic medicine going so far as to include daily preventive care of the oral cavity, nasal passages, sinuses, eyes and skin.

Alternative medical systems differ from conventional medicine in that treatments are individualized. No two individuals with similar symptoms receive the exact same treatment. For example, two women undergoing menopause and experiencing hot flashes who see a practitioner of traditional Chinese medicine could receive different forms of acupuncture therapy and different herbs depending on their individual "constitutional" diagnoses.

To date, research has generally focused on studying individual components of alternative medical systems and not the whole system, which is more complex. For example, there's research supporting the use of acupuncture in the management of osteoarthritis, postoperative nausea and vomiting. But acupuncture is only one component of traditional Chinese medicine. Likewise, there's research supporting the use of yoga for cancer fatigue and low back pain, but yoga is just one component of the ayurvedic system. Research on the effectiveness of whole medical systems is ongoing, and results are eagerly awaited.

Ayurveda

Ayurveda, which means "science of life," originated in India more than 5,000 years ago and is thought to be the world's oldest system of natural medicine.

The basic theories on which ayurvedic medicine is based are that all things in the universe are joined together and that all forms of life consist of combinations of three energy elements: wind, fire and water. When these elements are balanced, a person is healthy. When they're unbalanced, the body is weakened and susceptible to illness.

To restore harmony and balance and treat illness, some of the therapies used by ayurvedic practitioners include:

- Enemas, fasting, or use of certain foods or metals to eliminate impurities and cleanse the body
- Breathing exercises, herbs or certain foods to reduce symptoms
- Massage of the body's "vital points" where life energy is stored to reduce pain, lessen fatigue or improve circulation
- Nurturing therapies such as yoga and meditation to reduce worry and anxiety and promote balance and harmony

In India, ayurvedic medicine is still practiced by the majority of the population, although it exists side by side with conventional Western medicine.

Our take

Some treatments used in ayurvedic medicine, such as yoga, massage or meditation, appear to be safe and may be effective. There's likely little risk in giving them a try. However, good-quality scientific studies on ayurvedic practices are limited. Many therapies — especially those involving herbs or metals — lack sufficient scientific data to recommend their use. Researchers are investigating certain ayurvedic supplements, and more should be known about their effectiveness and safety within a few years. In the meantime, if you do use an ayurvedic supplement, do so only under a doctor's close supervision because some have the potential to be toxic.

What the research says

Ayurvedic practices are used to treat a wide variety of conditions and symptoms. Here's what some studies have found:

Cardiovascular disease

The herbal and mineral formulation abana may reduce the frequency and severity of angina pain, improve cardiac function and reduce high blood pressure. A type of bark powder called terminalia (arjuna) may be an effective anti-angina agent. Two modern formulations of traditional ayurvedic herbal remedies (MAK-4 and MAK-5) may be useful in preventing atherosclerosis.

Cognitive function

The herb brahmi may improve memory and cognitive function, and the herbal formula MAK-4 may enhance attention capacity.

Diabetes

Studies of ayurvedic remedies for treatment of diabetes have produced mixed or modest results.

Hepatitis

Results of one study suggests the herbal preparation Kamalahar may improve liver function. Root powder from the herb *Picrorhiza kurroa* may also be effective.

Osteoarthritis

A study of a formula containing roots of *Withania somnifera*, the stem of *Boswellia serrata*, rhizomes of *Curcuma longa* and zinc complex found it may improve arthritis symptoms.

Body elements

Ayurvedic medicine is based on some specific beliefs as to how the body functions.

Prana

An important concept of ayurvedic medicine is that the human body houses a vital life energy called *prana*. Prana — similar to "qi" in traditional Chinese medicine and "ki" in traditional Japanese medicine — is the basis of life and healing.

Doshas

As this vital life energy circulates throughout the body, it's influenced by elements called *doshas*. Doshas control the basic activities of the body, and they formulate important individual characteristics.

Each dosha is composed of a combination of basic elements: space (ether), air, fire, water and earth. These elements represent subtle qualities of life energy and how the energy expresses itself within the body.

Doshas are influenced by diet, activity and body processes and are continuously being formulated and reformulated. An imbalance in a particular dosha will produce symptoms related to that dosha, which are different from symptoms produced by an imbalance in another dosha.

Prakriti

Certain doshas are predominant in each individual and determine that person's "constitution." The ayurvedic term for constitution is *prakriti*.

Your constitution refers to your general health, how likely your body is to become out of balance, and your body's ability to resist or recover from illness.

Ayurvedic belief is that your constitution does not change over your lifetime.

The details on doshas

There are three main doshas. Each person has his or her own unique balance of the three, although one dosha is usually predominant.

- **Vata dosha.** The vata dosha is a combination of the elements of space and air. It's considered the most powerful dosha because it controls movement and essential body processes such as cell division, the heart, breathing and the mind. The vata dosha can be thrown off balance by things such as staying up late at night or eating before the previous meal is digested. People with vata as their main dosha are thought to be especially susceptible to skin, neurological and mental illnesses.

- **Pitta dosha.** The pitta dosha is a combination of the elements of fire and water. The pitta dosha is believed to control the body's hormones and digestive system. When the pitta dosha is out of balance, a person may experience negative emotions, such as anger or jealousy, or digestive symptoms, such as heartburn. The pitta dosha can be thrown off balance by eating spicy or sour food, by being angry, tired or fearful, or by spending too much time in the sun. People with pitta as their main dosha are thought to be susceptible to heart disease and arthritis.

- **Kapha dosha.** The kapha dosha combines the elements of water and earth. The kapha dosha is thought to help maintain strength and immunity and control growth. When the kapha dosha is out of balance, a person may experience nausea immediately after eating. Napping during the day, eating too many sweets, eating after you're full, and eating and drinking too many foods and beverages with too much salt and water also may aggravate the kapha dosha. People with kapha as their main dosha are thought to be vulnerable to diabetes, gallbladder problems, stomach ulcers and respiratory illnesses.

Homeopathy

Homeopathy is a form of health care developed in Germany, which has been practiced in the United States since the early 19th century.

A key premise of homeopathic medicine is that every person has a form of energy called a vital force, or self-healing response. When this force is disrupted or out of balance, illness results.

Homeopathy aims to stimulate the body's healing response. Treatment generally involves giving very small doses of substances called remedies. These remedies are formulated according to two beliefs:

- **The law of similars.** When given to a healthy person in large quantities, some plant, animal and mineral substances produce symptoms of disease. But when given to a sick person, much smaller doses of the same substances can (theoretically) relieve the same symptoms. This theory is sometimes referred to as "like cures like."

- **The law of infinitesimals.** Infinitesimal means too small to be measured. The belief is substances treat disease most effectively when they're highly diluted (often distilled in water or alcohol) to the point where none of the original substance remains.

Homeopathic remedies are sold in liquid, tablet and pellet forms. Treatment may also include changes in diet, exercise and other lifestyle behaviors.

Our take

Homeopathic medicine is popular. However, it lacks good studies to prove its effectiveness. Studies that have been done have generally been small and have produced conflicting results. In general, the scientific community also finds the theories on which homeopathic medicine is based questionable and difficult to accept. These factors have kept it from being widely accepted into mainstream medicine.

Because homeopathic medicine mainly involves diluted substances containing little, if any, of their original formulas, the risk they pose is likely minimal. The risks you may be taking is the money you spend if it doesn't work, or if you forgo proven conventional treatments for homeopathic therapies.

What the research says

Few, if any, studies on homeopathy as a whole — a complete system of medicine — have been published. Some studies on specific treatments have been conducted, but they've been small or the quality and accuracy of the studies have been questioned. More research is needed before any recommendations can be made:

Acute childhood diarrhea

Studies suggest homeopathic treatment may improve digestion and decrease duration of acute diarrhea episodes in children.

Allergies

For treatment of hay fever, one study found a homeopathic nasal spray may be as effective as the conventional spray cromolyn sodium. For treatment of perennial allergic rhinitis, one study found a homeopathic preparation may improve nasal airflow.

Influenza

The homeopathic remedy oscillococcinum has been studied as a possible treatment to reduce the duration of flu symptoms.

Pain

Homeopathic approaches to treat pain, including arthritic pain, show some promise but the evidence is preliminary.

Vertigo

Homeopathic therapies may work as well as conventional treatment in people with vertigo.

Naturopathy

Naturopathy is a form of health care based on the belief that the body has an innate healing power that can establish, maintain and restore health when it's in a healthy environment.

Naturopathic medicine relies on natural remedies, such as sunlight, air and water, along with "natural" supplements to promote health and well-being.

Based on their belief in the healing power of nature, early naturopaths often prescribed hydrotherapy — soaks in hot springs and other water-related therapies — to treat illness. Today, naturopathic practitioners draw on many forms of complementary and alternative medicine, including practices such as massage, acupuncture, exercise and lifestyle counseling.

In addition to the body's natural ability to heal, practitioners of naturopathy believe that healing should come in the most gentle, least invasive and most efficient manner possible.

Individuals who provide naturopathic care aren't all the same. A naturopath is a therapist who practices naturopathy. A naturopathic physician is a primary health care provider trained in a broad scope of naturopathic practices in addition to a standard medical curriculum. Both use the designation of N.D. — representing either naturopathic diploma or naturopathic doctor — which can cause confusion about the person's scope of practice, education and training.

Our take

Much of the advice of naturopaths is worth heeding: exercise regularly, practice good nutrition, quit smoking and enjoy nature. However, claims that treatments such as hydrotherapy detoxify the body and strengthen the immune system aren't backed up by scientific research. And just because a product or practice is considered "natural" doesn't mean it's safe.

Some aspects of naturopathic medicine may be used to complement conventional medical treatment. But be wary of naturopathic practitioners who recommend that you avoid prescription drugs or surgery or other treatments known to be beneficial.

What the research says

Similar to homeopathy, there haven't been any quality research studies conducted on naturopathy as a whole — a complete system of medicine. There's no evidence that naturopathic medicine can cure cancer or any other disease, as some proponents claim.

A limited number of studies have been done on herbs used as naturopathic treatments. One study found that echinacea wasn't effective in treating colds in children, while another suggested an herbal extract containing echinacea may reduce ear pain associated with ear infections (acute otitis media). A study of another multi-ingredient naturopathic extract also indicated possible benefits in reducing ear pain associated with ear infection.

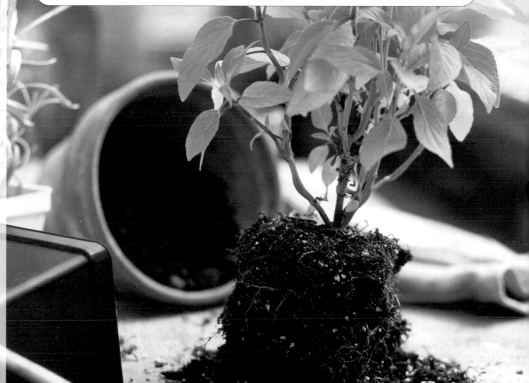

Traditional Chinese medicine

Traditional Chinese medicine is a system of medicine rooted in ancient Chinese philosophy (Taoism).

Traditional Chinese medicine is based on the belief that the body is a delicate balance of two opposing forces: yin and yang. Yin represents the cold, slow or passive principle of life, while yang represents the hot, excited, active one. Health is achieved by maintaining an appropriate balance of the two.

An imbalance of yin and yang leads to blockage in the flow of blood and vital life energy (qi) along pathways known as meridians. To help unblock these pathways and restore health, practitioners of traditional Chinese medicine generally use one or a combination of treatments, which may include:

- Acupuncture, moxibustion or cupping
- Chinese herbs
- Massage and manipulation
- Qi gong (see page 109)

Moxibustion is the application of heat from burning of the herb moxa at an acupuncture point. Cupping involves placing a heated cup over a part of the body. As the air inside cools, its volume decreases, creating a slight suction and stimulating blood flow.

Chinese herbs are usually processed as pills, capsules or powders — but the raw, dried forms common centuries ago are still used. There are more than 2,000 Chinese herbs.

Our take

In China, traditional Chinese medicine is integrated into the country's health care system and used side by side with modern medicine. In the United States we generally pick and choose certain components of traditional Chinese medicine and use them in isolation. Practices such as acupuncture, massage and manipulation can be of benefit in treating certain conditions. A few Chinese herbs also may be of use in treating conditions such as cardiovascular disease and side effects of cancer. However, Chinese herbs need to be approached with caution. They can be very powerful, and some are dangerous. Ephedra (ma-huang), the main active ingredient in many "natural" weight-loss products, is thought to have caused 22 deaths and 800 cases of toxicity.

What the research says

The individual component within traditional Chinese medicine that has received the most study is acupuncture. For more information on acupuncture, see page 106. For information on Chinese massage (tui na), see page 119. As for Chinese herbs, only a few good studies have been conducted. A challenge is that most Chinese herbs are used in combination, not alone.

Autoimmune and inflammatory disease

A small randomized trial of the Chinese herb thunder god vine showed a positive response in people with rheumatoid arthritis. A larger study found it to cause renal, cardiac and other toxicities.

Cancer

Studies suggest Chinese herbs may shrink tumors, reduce side effects and improve response to treatment. But the quality of the studies has been weak. Better studies are needed.

Cardiovascular disease

Chinese herb formulas are taken to reduce symptoms of angina, stabilize abnormal heart rhythms, and improve heart function and blood composition. While there's some evidence of potential benefits, the studies have been limited and of poor design.

Menopausal symptoms

Chinese herbs are used to treat symptoms of menopause. They may benefit memory, but don't seem to improve hot flashes.

The human 'ecosystem'

According to ancient Chinese belief, the laws that govern the natural world also apply to human life. A person is viewed as an individual ecosystem, related to a larger ecosystem.

The goal of traditional Chinese medicine is to maintain natural harmony. Harmony and disharmony — health and sickness — are determined according to concepts known as principles, elements and networks.

These concepts are all taken into consideration in determining the cause of illness and how to treat it.

8 principles

The eight principles are actually four pairs of opposites that describe patterns of disharmony.

- Interior/exterior refers to the location of the disharmony in the body — internal organs vs. skin or bones.
- Hot/cold refers to the symptoms of the disease, such as fever or thirst vs. chilliness or the desire to drink something warm.
- Full/empty refers to whether the condition is acute or chronic, and whether the body's responses are strong or weak.
- The balance of yin/yang — the cold, passive principle of life vs. the hot, active one — is also a factor in determining disharmony and identifying disease.

5 elements

The five elements are: fire, earth, metal, water and wood. The terms refer to dynamic qualities of nature and describe changes in the flow of life energy.

The five elements build upon one another and mutually reinforce each other. If one is out of balance, it can impair another.

The elements follow this sequence: wood creates fire, fire creates earth, earth creates metal, metal creates water and water creates wood.

5 networks

The body has five organ networks that each respond to a particular element:
- Heart/small intestine with fire
- Spleen/stomach with earth
- Lungs/large intestine with metal
- Kidneys/bladder with water
- Liver/gallbladder with wood

Acupressure: Benefits of putting on the pressure

Acupressure is a traditional Chinese medicine technique based on the same ideas as acupuncture. It involves placing physical pressure at specific points on the surface of the body by means of a finger, hand, elbow or various devices. The intent is to restore the flow of life energy (qi). Another term for acupressure is *shiatsu*.

Acupressure is used to treat a wide variety of conditions including musculoskeletal pain and tension, depression, anxiety, sleep difficulties, headache and nausea. Some people also use it as a relaxation technique.

One condition for which studies have shown acupressure to be effective is in treating nausea. Numerous scientific studies support the use of acupressure applied to a specific point (P6) on the wrist to prevent and treat nausea associated with surgery and chemotherapy, as well as nausea related to morning sickness that accompanies pregnancy. Some people have also found wrist acupressure effective in reducing motion sickness.

The P6 point is located about three finger-widths from the large crease in your wrist (see illustration).

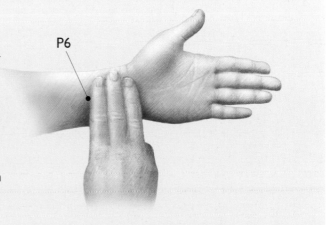

P6

Part 3

Your Action Plan

Choosing the best treatments for better health

The guiding philosophy of today's "new medicine" — integrative medicine — is to blend the best of complementary and conventional therapies to treat the whole person, not just the disease.

In Part 3, we take a look at 20 common conditions and offer advice on treatment and prevention, combining nontraditional therapies with conventional care to achieve optimal health.

We also discuss important information regarding safety. Complementary and alternative practices aren't regulated in the same manner as are prescription medications and other forms of conventional care. Therefore, it's important to be smart in how you approach complementary and alternative medicine, and not be fooled by fraudulent claims.

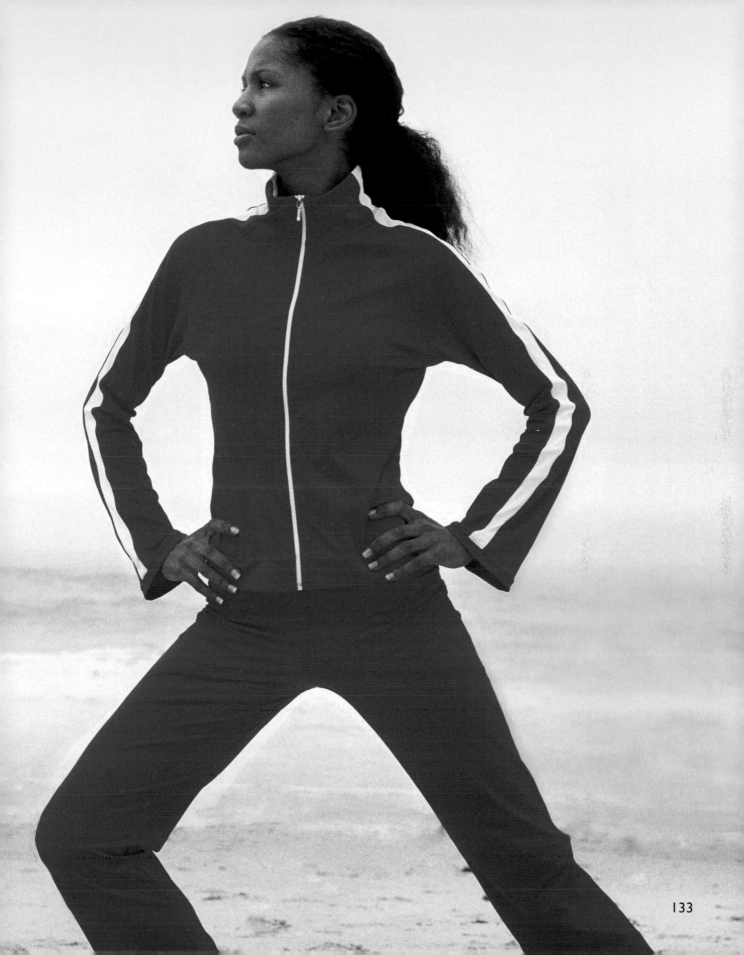

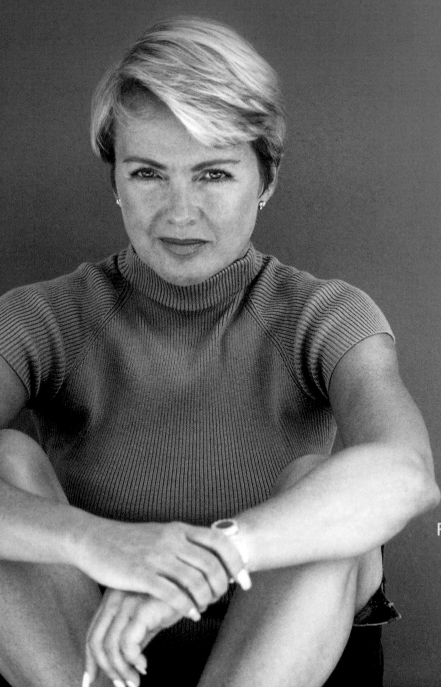

Chapter 8
Treating 20 Common Conditions

A visit with Dr. Dietlind Wahner-Roedler

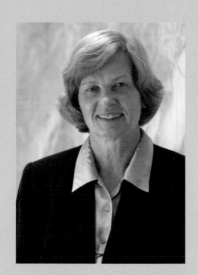

Dietlind Wahner-Roedler, M.D.
General Internal Medicine

" *The challenge for the coming decade will be to sift the 'wheat from the chaff' — incorporating those products and practices that are effective and safe, while avoiding those that aren't.* "

For much of the latter part of the 20th century, conventional medicine made amazing strides, from conquering polio to developing microscopic surgical techniques. It seemed that advancing research might be all that was needed to eradicate disease. In such a world, it's not surprising that some people took a casual approach to their health. After all, if smoking and poor diet led to a heart attack, medicine had a ready fix in bypass surgery or better yet, a stent. Why take the time to invest in your health if modern medicine could alleviate the consequences of bad choices? Unfortunately, modern medicine doesn't have all the answers.

What we've seen in today's medicine is a fabulous ability to "fix" things, once they're "broken" — treating heart attacks with coronary artery bypass surgery, kidney failure with kidney transplant or obesity with bariatric surgery. Yet the same degree of emphasis and expertise hasn't developed in regard to preventing these problems. Nor has as much focus been given to steps people can take when faced with a chronic condition that isn't amenable to a quick fix — such as high blood pressure, diabetes and arthritis. With the rapid aging of the U.S. population, it is becoming evident that self-care may be more important now than ever before.

Much of complementary and alternative medicine is focused on prevention — a heavy emphasis on diet, physical activity, stress reduction and maintaining connectedness — and on dealing with chronic issues more effectively. This might include using yoga in addition to medication to treat high blood pressure, or trying cinnamon in addition to dietary changes to control high blood sugar. Sometimes, alternative medicine is a replacement to conventional medicine when a proven treatment isn't feasible because of side effects. An example is use of nonsteroidal anti-inflammatory drugs (NSAIDs) to treat arthritis. Though they control pain, they can also cause ulcers or high blood pressure.

The difficulty incorporating more complementary and alternative therapies into the current health care regimen is that collective experience and knowledge regarding how to safely integrate such treatments is still largely in its infancy. While research is growing rapidly in this area, limited regulatory control has allowed ineffective and even dangerous alternatives to reach mass markets. The challenge for the coming decade will be to sift the "wheat from the chaff" — incorporating those products and practices that are effective and safe, while avoiding those that aren't.

To help with this challenge, the following chapter focuses on 20 common conditions and their conventional and complementary treatments. We look at the evidence for and against the most commonly encountered alternative treatments, giving recommendations where the evidence is strongest and more cautionary notes when the evidence is less or the risk is high. By following the same approach with other conditions as is outlined in these examples, you should be able to develop a sound approach to evaluating new therapies as they arise.

Arthritis

When you think of arthritis, you likely think of pain and stiffness in joints. And you'd be right on the money. Those are typical symptoms of osteoarthritis and rheumatoid arthritis, the two most common forms of arthritis (there are actually more than 100 forms).

Arthritis is the leading cause of disability in the United States. In fact, more than one-fourth of U.S. adults report ongoing pain or stiffness in their joints, and more than 45 million Americans have been diagnosed with some form of arthritis.

Osteoarthritis is commonly known as wear-and-tear arthritis. It involves the wearing away of the tough, lubricated cartilage that normally cushions the ends of bones in your joints. Rheumatoid arthritis results from an abnormal immune system response that causes inflammation of the lining of the joints.

Arthritis affects people of all ages, but it's most common among older adults. Women, possibly because of female hormones, are at higher risk of many forms of arthritis than are men.

Whites, blacks and American Indians are more likely to get arthritis than are Asians and Hispanics. In addition, people who are more than 10 pounds overweight are at increased risk, especially of arthritis of the knees. Past joint injury also can increase risk of osteoarthritis.

Conventional Treatment for Osteoarthritis

There's no known cure for osteoarthritis, but treatments can help to reduce pain and maintain joint movement. Conventional treatment typically involves a combination of therapies that may include medication, self-care, physical therapy and occupational therapy. In some cases, surgical procedures may be necessary.

Medications

Medications are used to treat the pain and mild inflammation of osteoarthritis and to improve the function of your joints. They include both topical medications and oral medications. Nonprescription topical pain relievers include Aspercreme, Sportscreme, Icy Hot, Ben-Gay, and various formulations containing capsaicin, a cream made from hot chili (cayenne) peppers.

Nonprescription medications such as acetaminophen (Tylenol, others), aspirin, ibuprofen (Advil, Motrin IB, others) and naproxen sodium (Aleve) may be sufficient to treat milder osteoarthritis, but stronger prescription medications also are available. These include the COX-2 inhibitor celecoxib (Celebrex), tramadol (Ultram) and various antidepressants.

Occasionally, your doctor may suggest injecting a joint space with a corticosteroid to relieve pain and swelling. Injecting hyaluronic acid derivatives into knee joints (viscosupplementation) also can relieve pain from osteoarthritis.

Surgical or other procedures

Surgical procedures can help relieve disability and pain caused by osteoarthritis. Procedures include joint replacement, arthroscopic lavage and debridement to remove debris from a joint, bone repositioning to help correct deformities, and bone fusion to increase stability and reduce pain.

Self-care

Fortunately, you can relieve much of the discomfort associated with osteoarthritis through healthy-living strategies and self-care techniques.

These include exercising regularly to maintain mobility and range of motion, controlling your weight to reduce stress on joints, eating a healthy diet (to help control your weight), applying heat to ease pain and relax tense, painful muscles, and applying cold to dull the sensation of occasional flare-ups.

In addition, choosing comfortable, cushioned footwear is important if you have arthritis in your weight-bearing joints or back. And, it's important to take your medications as recommended to keep pain from increasing.

Complementary & Alternative Treatment

There appears to be relatively good evidence that several complementary and alternative therapies can help relieve the pain of osteoarthritis.

Common therapies

Glucosamine and chondroitin. Glucosamine sulfate is a dietary supplement derived from oyster and crab shells. It's a synthetic version of an amino sugar the body produces to preserve joint health. Chondroitin sulfate is a dietary supplement derived from cow and shark cartilage and other sources. The two are often used in combination.

Glucosamine may reduce pain and joint tenderness as effectively as do nonsteroidal anti-inflammatory drugs (NSAIDs), such as aspirin and ibuprofen (Advil, Motrin IB, others). Chondroitin may reduce pain over time, and when used with NSAIDs can relieve pain and improve hip and knee function. A large study completed in 2005 found that, compared with a placebo, the combination of glucosamine and chondroitin produced some reduction in pain for people with more severe osteoarthritic symptoms. It was less effective for mild pain. The supplements can cause mild gastrointestinal effects but generally produce fewer side effects than do NSAIDs. Don't take glucosamine if you're allergic to shellfish.

Acupuncture. Research indicates that acupuncture may relieve pain from osteoarthritis in some individuals, especially knee pain. It's generally a low-risk treatment. Find an experienced practitioner.

SAM-e. Commercially available SAM-e is a synthetic version of a compound that occurs naturally in human tissue. The dietary supplement appears to relieve pain from osteoarthritis as effectively as NSAIDs but with fewer side effects. You may need to take SAM-e for up to a month before you experience significant relief from symptoms.

Side effects can include flatulence, vomiting, diarrhea, headache and nausea. SAM-e can negatively interact with antidepressant medications.

Relaxation techniques. Techniques such as hypnosis, relaxed breathing, guided imagery and muscle relaxation may help to control pain.

Avocado extract. It may help with symptoms of osteoarthritis and is generally considered safe. Use caution if you're sensitive to latex. Safety of the combination of avocado and soybean oil needs long-term study.

Devil's claw. This herb may reduce pain from osteoarthritis and generally appears safe. It may not be safe for people with gastric or heart problems, or for children or pregnant or lactating women.

Little evidence

Although they remain popular, there's little evidence to support use of magnets for arthritis. On the plus side, side effects appear rare. But, magnets can disrupt pacemakers and may harm the baby during pregnancy.

Coping skills are important

Because osteoarthritis can affect your everyday activities and overall quality of life, coping strategies are an important element of dealing with the disease, whether you choose conventional or alternative treatments.

Coping strategies include keeping a positive attitude so you're in charge of your disease, rather than vice versa, knowing when to limit activities, using assistive devices, and avoiding grasping actions that can strain finger joints.

Strategies also include spreading the weight of an object over several joints when lifting, such as using both hands to lift a heavy pan, maintaining good posture to evenly distribute your weight, and using your strongest muscles and large joints (for example, leaning into a heavy door to open it rather than pushing it with your hands).

An occupational therapist can also help you in selecting the right assistive devices for daily living.

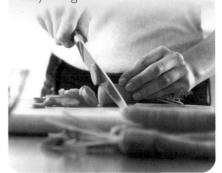

Conventional Treatment for Rheumatoid Arthritis

Treatment typically involves a combination of self-care techniques similar to those used for osteoarthritis (see page 136) and medications. Sometimes, surgery or other procedures may be necessary.

Medication

Medications for rheumatoid arthritis can relieve its symptoms and slow or halt its progression. Medications used include nonsteroidal anti-inflammatory drugs (NSAIDs), such as aspirin and ibuprofen (Advil, Motrin IB, others), the COX-2 inhibitor celecoxib (Celebrex), corticosteroids, such as prednisone and methylprednisolone (Medrol), and disease-modifying antirheumatic drugs (DMARDs), such as hydroxychloroquine (Plaquenil) and methotrexate (Rheumatrex).

Also used are immunosuppressants, such as leflunomide (Arava) and azathioprine (Imuran), TNF blockers, such as etanercept (Enbrel) and infliximab (Remicade), the interleukin-1 receptor antagonist anakinra (Kineret), and the drugs abatacept (Orencia) and rituximab (Rituxan).

Surgery and other procedures

If joint destruction is too severe, joint replacement can often help restore joint function, reduce pain or correct a deformity.

Complementary & Alternative Treatment

Evidence appears strongest that fish oil supplements offer the most promise as an integrative treatment.

Common therapies

Omega-3 fatty acids. Research shows that regularly taking omega-3 fatty acid (fish oil) supplements for up to three months can improve morning stiffness and joint tenderness in people with rheumatoid arthritis. But the effect of the supplements has not been well studied beyond three months. Because high doses can cause bleeding, don't take more than 3 grams (3,000 milligrams) a day without consulting a doctor.

Conflicting or unclear evidence

Among other therapies, boswellia, cat's claw, evening primrose oil and ginger fall into the uncertain category. Cat's claw may produce modest benefits. Evening primrose oil and ginger are likely safe in small quantities. Boswellia may be as well, except for pregnant women, as it may induce abortion. In addition, the Indian spice turmeric has been shown in lab studies to have anti-inflammatory properties, but its use in treating rheumatoid arthritis remains uncertain. All need more study.

Chronic fatigue syndrome

Chronic fatigue syndrome (CFS) is a complicated disorder characterized by extreme fatigue that doesn't improve with bed rest and may worsen with physical or mental activity.

Of all chronic illnesses, chronic fatigue syndrome is one of the most mysterious. Unlike infections, it has no clear cause. Unlike conditions such as diabetes or anemia, there's essentially nothing to measure. And unlike conditions such as heart disease, there are relatively few treatment options.

Chronic fatigue syndrome may occur after an infection such as a cold or viral syndrome. It can start during or shortly after a period of high stress or come on gradually without any clear starting point or any obvious cause. Chronic fatigue syndrome is a flu-like condition that can drain your energy and sometimes last for years. People previously healthy and full of energy may experience a variety of symptoms, including extreme fatigue, weakness and headaches as well as difficulty concentrating and painful joints, muscles and lymph nodes.

Women are diagnosed with chronic fatigue syndrome two to four times as often as are men. However, it's unclear whether chronic fatigue syndrome affects women more frequently or if women report it to their doctors more often than do men.

Conventional Treatment

There's no specific conventional treatment for chronic fatigue syndrome. In general, doctors aim to relieve symptoms by using a combination of treatments, which may include:

Lifestyle changes. Your doctor may encourage you to slow down and to avoid excessive physical and psychological stress. This may save your energy for essential activities at home or work and help you cut back on less important activities.

Gradual but steady exercise. Often, with the help of a physical therapist, you may be advised to begin a graduated exercise program in which physical activity gradually increases. This can help prevent or decrease the muscle weakness caused by prolonged inactivity. In addition, your energy level can often improve significantly.

Treatment of psychiatric problems. Doctors can treat problems often related to chronic fatigue syndrome, such as depression, with medication or behavior therapy — learning to change your behavior to reduce the symptoms of a certain disease or condition — or a combination of the two. If you're depressed, medications such as tricyclic antidepressants and selective serotonin reuptake inhibitors (SSRIs) may help. Even if you are not depressed, antidepressants may still help improve sleep and relieve pain. Tricyclic antidepressants include amitriptyline (Limbitrol — a multi-ingredient drug that contains amitriptyline), desipramine (Norpramin) and nortriptyline (Aventyl, Pamelor). SSRIs include fluoxetine (Prozac, Sarafem), paroxetine (Paxil), sertraline (Zoloft) and bupropion (Wellbutrin).

Treatment of existing pain. Acetaminophen (Tylenol, others) or nonsteroidal anti-inflammatory drugs (NSAIDs) such as aspirin and ibuprofen (Advil, Motrin IB, others) may be helpful to reduce pain and fever.

Treatment of allergy-like symptoms. Antihistamines such as fexofenadine (Allegra) and cetirizine (Zyrtec) and decongestants that contain pseudoephedrine (Sudafed, Dimetapp) may relieve allergy-like symptoms such as runny nose.

Treatment of low blood pressure (hypotension). The drugs fludrocortisone (Florinef), atenolol (Tenormin) and midodrine (ProAmatine) may be useful for certain people with chronic fatigue syndrome who have an unusual blood pressure response.

Some medications can cause side effects or adverse reactions that may be worse than the symptoms of chronic fatigue syndrome. Talk to your doctor before starting any treatment for this condition.

Complementary & Alternative Treatment

Because the causes of chronic fatigue syndrome are not clear, an integrative approach to treatment involves addressing a variety of possible factors. These include diet, hormone balances, underlying infections, insomnia, pain and dysfunction of the body's energy-production system.

Diet. Poor dietary habits and nutrient deficiencies can lead to fatigue. Avoiding simple sugars and foods with a high glycemic index, such as white flour and potatoes, may help eliminate large fluctuations in blood sugar levels that can be associated with fatigue. Avoiding caffeine and addressing nutritional deficiencies such as low iron stores also may help.

Hormone balances. In addition to considering conventional therapies for hormone problems, an integrative approach might look at, for example, use of such alternative treatments as licorice, vitamin C or ginseng for adrenal issues. Licorice, however, may make heartburn symptoms worse, and high doses of vitamin C can cause loose stools. Ginseng can be stimulating and may worsen insomnia.

Underlying infections. Some complementary and alternative practitioners believe that people with chronic fatigue syndrome may be experiencing chronic infections, especially yeast infections and chronic sinusi-

tis. Alternative treatment of a yeast infection might include use of probiotics, such as eating live-culture yogurt (see page 82). For chronic sinusitis, alternative treatment might include nasal irrigation with a neti pot (see page 157).

Insomnia. Although people with chronic fatigue syndrome are fatigued, many report difficulty sleeping. In addition to considering conventional sleep medications, an integrative approach might consider melatonin, valerian, passionflower or calcium and magnesium at bedtime. Some people, though, find valerian overstimulating rather than sleep-inducing.

Pain. An integrative approach to pain management might include — in addition to conventional therapies — massage, yoga, therapy to improve posture problems, and acupuncture. Herbal approaches might include the use of cayenne or glucosamine and chondroitin for joint pain.

Energy. Fatigue could indicate a problem at the cellular level where the chemical reaction that releases energy takes place. Alternative approaches might include use of potassium and magnesium, if deficiencies exist, coenzyme Q10, carnitine in the form of acetyl-L, and lysine, and vitamin C and B vitamins if there are deficiencies.

Primary signs and symptoms of CFS

In addition to persistent fatigue not caused by other known medical conditions, chronic fatigue syndrome has eight possible primary signs and symptoms. These include:

- Loss of memory or concentration
- Sore throat
- Painful and mildly enlarged lymph nodes in your neck or armpits (axillae)
- Unexplained muscle soreness
- Pain that moves from one joint to another without swelling or redness
- Headache of a new type, pattern or severity
- Sleep disturbance
- Extreme exhaustion after normal exercise or exertion

According to a Centers for Disease Control and Prevention (CDC) study group, a person meets the diagnostic criteria of chronic fatigue syndrome when unexplained persistent fatigue occurs for six months or more with at least four of the eight primary signs and symptoms also present.

Chronic pain

If you have a condition such as a broken bone, you recognize discomfort as a symptom and trust that treatment will help. After surgery, pain medication provides relief while your body heals. Chronic pain is different.

Sometimes, chronic pain follows an illness or an injury that appears to have healed. It can also be related to long-standing conditions such as arthritis. Other times, chronic pain develops for no apparent reason.

Whatever the cause, the emotional fallout of chronic pain can make you hurt even more. Anxiety or depression can magnify unpleasant sensations, and disrupted sleep may leave you feeling fatigued and helpless.

Conventional Treatment

Chronic pain is a challenge, but there are a variety of conventional treatment options. They include:

Medication. Sometimes, over-the-counter pain relievers or medicated creams or gels are effective. For more severe pain, your doctor may prescribe an opioid medication. Some people find relief with tricyclic antidepressants such as nortriptyline (Pamelor). Seizure drugs such as gabapentin (Neurontin) or carbamazepine (Tegretol) may relieve some types of chronic pain as well.

Injection therapy. Instead of prescribing pills to control chronic pain, your doctor might inject medication directly into the affected area. Such injections are usually a combination of a numbing agent (local anesthetic), which provides immediate relief, and a corticosteroid, which reduces inflammation.

Nerve stimulation. Various devices use electric impulses to help block or mask the feeling of pain. With transcutaneous electrical nerve stimulation (TENS), a portable, battery-powered unit delivers an electric impulse through electrodes placed on the affected area. Spinal cord and peripheral nerve stimulators are implanted beneath the skin with electrodes placed near the spinal cord. A hand-held unit allows you to control the level of stimulation.

Medication pumps. An implantable medication pump supplies pain medication directly into the spinal fluid. To replenish the pump, drugs are injected through the skin into a small port at the center of the pump.

Physical and occupational therapy. Stretching and strengthening exercises can improve your strength and flexibility. Sometimes learning new ways to handle daily activities can minimize the pain.

Counseling. A counselor can help you manage your emotional response to chronic pain, as well as identify patterns of thought or behavior that may aggravate your pain.

Exercise. Exercise can prompt your body to release endorphins, chemicals that block pain signals from reaching your brain. It can also help you build strength, increase flexibility, improve sleep quality and boost your energy level. In addition, it can improve mood and protect your heart and blood vessels. If you have chronic pain, talk to your doctor before starting an exercise program.

Complementary & Alternative Treatment

Various complementary therapies, including acupuncture, guided imagery, hypnosis and music therapy, may offer relief from chronic pain.

Common therapies

Acupuncture. This traditional Chinese therapy involves the insertion of fine needles into the skin at certain points to restore proper energy flow in the body. Research indicates that it may relieve pain from osteoarthritis, especially knee pain. It's generally a low-risk treatment, but use of unsterilized needles can result in infection. Find an experienced practitioner.

Guided imagery. This can refer to a number of therapies, including visualization, game-playing and storytelling. The goal is to help people visualize positive outcomes for issues they're dealing with. Guided imagery may alter breathing, heart rate and blood pressure. With pain, it's been shown to reduce postoperative pain and pain from laparoscopic surgery. It may also reduce cancer pain. Guided imagery is generally considered safe. However, theoretically it could interact with certain mental conditions, so use it only with professional guidance if you have mental health issues.

Hypnosis. Hypnosis involves inducing a deep state of relaxation that opens the participant to suggestion. How it actually works is not known, but it can affect heart rate, blood pressure and body temperature. There's strong evidence that hypnosis can reduce chronic pain associated with cancer. It may also help with chronic pain from irritable bowel syndrome, tension headaches and certain other conditions.

There is no universal certification standard for hypnotists in the United States. Safety concerns are similar for those with guided imagery.

Music therapy. Music can influence your physical and emotional states. Music therapists are trained to adapt the therapy to meet specific needs of individuals. It's been shown to raise pain thresholds, improve mood and provide relaxation, and has been effective in reducing pain from cancer, burns, osteoarthritis and surgery, among other conditions.

Conflicting or unclear evidence

In healing (therapeutic) touch, practitioners hold their hands close to a person to supposedly sense and manipulate the person's energy field. There's very little proof that it actually works, but many people report that they feel very relaxed after a healing touch session. Pending more studies, it falls into the category of "may not help but probably doesn't hurt."

Similarly, magnet therapy is popular but has very little in the way of scientific evidence to support its use as a pain treatment. Risks are mostly financial — although magnetic bracelets can cost only a few dollars, mattresses can cost hundreds or thousands of dollars.

Back pain

The back is a well-designed structure made up of bone, muscles, nerves and other soft tissues. You rely on your back to be the workhorse of the body — its function is essential for nearly every move you make. Because of this, the back can be particularly vulnerable to injury and back pain can be disabling.

Four out of five adults have at least one bout of back pain sometime during life. In fact, back pain is one of the most common reasons for health care visits and missed work.

On the bright side, you can prevent most back pain. Simple home treatment and proper body mechanics will often heal your back within a few weeks and keep it functional for the long haul. Surgery is rarely needed to treat back pain.

Treating back pain

Most back pain gets better with a few weeks of home treatment and careful attention. A regular schedule of pain relievers and hot or cold therapy may be all that you need. A short period of bed rest is OK, but more than a couple of days actually does more harm than good. If home treatments aren't working, your doctor may suggest:

Physical therapy and exercise. A physical therapist can apply treatments, such as heat, ice, ultrasound, electrical stimulation and muscle release techniques, to back muscles and soft tissues to reduce pain.

Prescription medications. Your doctor may prescribe nonsteroidal anti-inflammatory drugs or in some cases, a muscle relaxant.

Cortisone injections. For pain from a "pinched nerve," your doctor may prescribe cortisone injections — an anti-inflammatory medication — into the space around your spinal cord (epidural space).

Electrical stimulation. Transcutaneous electrical nerve stimulation (TENS) uses a unit that sends a weak electrical current through points on the skin to nerve pathways. This is thought to interrupt pain signals.

Back schools. These programs, available in many communities, focus on managing back pain and preventing its recurrence.

Additional treatments. For chronic back pain, treatment may also include antidepressant medications, which can relieve pain independent of their effect on depression, opioid medications, such as codeine or hydrocodone, or medications administered through a pump.

Surgery. Few people ever need surgery for back pain. There are no effective surgical techniques for muscle- and soft-tissue-related back pain. Surgery is usually reserved for pain caused by a herniated disk.

Beyond the basics

Common complementary and alternative therapies include chiropractic manipulation, acupuncture, hydrotherapy and massage.

Chiropractic manipulation. Spinal adjustment may help uncomplicated low back pain, especially when performed shortly after the pain begins. Evidence doesn't support its use for severe back pain. Manipulation of the neck may be unsafe for people with vascular problems or an aneurysm. Use caution if you have osteoporosis.

Hydrotherapy. For low back pain, hot whirlpool baths, combined with standard therapy, may help. Be cautious of high temperatures, and avoid intense water jets if you have blood clots, bleeding disorders, fractures, open wounds, severe osteoporosis or are pregnant.

Massage. This is a relatively safe way to relax tense muscles and help ease pain. Avoid if you have phlebitis, deep vein thrombosis, open wounds, inflamed or infected tissue, or an infectious disease.

Other treatments. Benefits are unproved but risks appear low for meditation, yoga and devil's claw when used for back pain.

Common cold

A common cold is an infection of your upper respiratory tract. It's relatively harmless — but it sure doesn't feel that way when you have one. If it's not a runny nose, sore throat and a cough, it's watery eyes, sneezing and miserable congestion. Or maybe all of the above. In fact, because any one of more than 200 viruses can cause a common cold, symptoms tend to vary greatly.

Unfortunately, if you're like most adults, you're likely to have a common cold two to four times a year. Children, especially preschoolers, may have a common cold as many as eight to 10 times annually.

The good news is that you or your child should be feeling better in about a week. If symptoms aren't improving in that time, see your doctor to make sure you don't have a bacterial infection in your lungs, larynx, trachea, sinuses or ears.

Conventional Treatment

There's no cure for the common cold. Antibiotics are of no use against cold viruses, and over-the-counter cold preparations won't cure a common cold or make it go away any sooner. However, over-the-counter medications can relieve some symptoms.

For fever, sore throat and headache, try acetaminophen (Tylenol, others) or other mild pain relievers. Don't give aspirin to children, because it may have a role in causing Reye's syndrome, a rare but potentially fatal disease.

For runny nose and nasal congestion, you can take an antihistamine or decongestant. Don't use decongestant drops and sprays for more than a few days, though, because prolonged use can cause chronic inflammation of your mucous membranes. And don't give them to children under age 2. There's little evidence that they work in young children, and they may cause side effects.

Self-care for colds

You may not be able to cure your common cold, but you can make yourself as comfortable as possible. These tips may help:

Drink lots of fluids. Avoid alcohol, caffeine and cigarette smoke, which can cause dehydration and aggravate your symptoms.

Get some rest. Consider staying home from work if you have a fever or a bad cough, or are drowsy from medications. This will give you a chance to rest as well as reduce the chances that you'll infect others. Wear a mask when you have a cold if you live or work with someone with a chronic disease or compromised immune system.

Adjust your room's temperature and humidity. Keep your room warm, but not overheated. If the air is dry, a cool-mist humidifier or vaporizer can moisten the air and help ease congestion and coughing. Be sure to keep the humidifier clean to prevent the growth of bacteria and molds.

Soothe your throat. Gargling with warm salt water several times a day or drinking warm lemon water with honey may help soothe a sore throat and relieve a cough.

Use nasal drops. To help relieve nasal congestion, try saline nasal drops. They're available without a prescription and are effective, safe and nonirritating, even for children. To use them, instill several drops into one nostril, then immediately bulb suction that nostril. Repeat in the opposite nostril.

Try chicken soup. Generations of parents have spooned chicken soup into their sick children. Now scientists have put chicken soup to the test, discovering that it does seem to help relieve cold and flu symptoms in two ways. First, it acts as an anti-inflammatory agent by inhibiting the movement of neutrophils — immune system cells that participate in the body's inflammatory response. Second, it temporarily speeds up the movement of mucus through the nose, helping relieve congestion and limiting the amount of time viruses are in contact with nasal lining. Researchers at the University of Nebraska compared homemade chicken soup with canned versions and found that many, though not all, canned chicken soups worked just as well as soups made from scratch.

Complementary & Alternative Treatment

Alternative therapies for the common cold are as common as colds. A few may have some value with little risk at typically used doses.

Andrographis. This herb is a popular cold and influenza treatment in Scandinavia and has been used for centuries in Asia. Although independent studies are limited, research suggests that andrographis can reduce the duration and severity of symptoms when taken early in an upper respiratory infection — within 36 to 48 hours of the onset of symptoms.

It appears safe at standardized commercial doses, but allergic reactions have been noted at higher doses. In addition, it may not be safe in combination with blood sugar lowering drugs, as it might push blood levels too low. Safety for long-term use is unclear.

Vitamin C. There's mixed evidence for using vitamin C to treat a cold. There appear to be no benefits for cold prevention or treatment for most people. However, studies have shown a roughly 50 percent cold-prevention benefit for people in extreme circumstances, such as marathon runners and soldiers in subarctic training.

Vitamin C supplements are generally considered safe at recommended doses. Higher doses, especially over 2,000 milligrams a day, may be associated with nausea, diarrhea and kidney stones.

Echinacea. Studies of echinacea use for the common cold are mixed, and its effectiveness is unclear. It's generally considered safe, but allergic reactions have been noted, especially rashes in children. It may cause an allergic reaction if you're allergic to plants in the Asteraceae or Compositae family (daisies, marigolds, ragweed, chrysanthemums). There's also concern it may not be safe for people with immune system disorders.

Garlic. Although garlic has been used for a long time for the prevention and treatment of colds, scientific evidence on the subject is slim. Although generally considered safe in quantities found in food, garlic may cause an allergic reaction. It may also increase the risk of bleeding, especially if you're taking a blood-thinning medication, such as aspirin, warfarin (Coumadin) or heparin.

Nasal irrigation. This therapy is similar to the conventional use of nasal drops (see preceding page), but more aggressive. It's more commonly used for hay fever and is relatively low risk (see page 157).

When to seek medical advice

A common cold generally goes away in about a week, although it may not disappear as quickly as you'd like. If your signs and symptoms last longer than a week, you may have a more serious illness, such as the flu or pneumonia.

Seek medical attention if you have:
- Fever greater than 102 F
- High fever accompanied by achiness and fatigue
- Fever accompanied by sweating, chills and a cough with colored phlegm
- Symptoms that get worse instead of better

In general, children are more sick with a common cold than are adults and often experience complications such as ear infections. Your child doesn't need to see a doctor for a routine common cold, but you should seek medical attention right away if your child has any of these signs or symptoms:
- Fever of 103 F or higher, chills or sweating
- Fever that lasts more than 72 hours
- Vomiting or abdominal pain
- Unusual sleepiness
- Severe headache
- Difficulty breathing
- Persistent crying
- Ear pain

Coronary artery disease

How healthy are your coronary arteries? If you eat healthy foods, get physical activity every day and don't smoke, you're well on your way to preventing symptoms of coronary artery disease — a leading type of heart disease.

The coronary arteries supply your heart with blood, oxygen and nutrients. When blood flow through the coronary arteries becomes obstructed, it's known as coronary artery disease.

Coronary artery disease is caused by the gradual buildup of fatty deposits in your coronary arteries (atherosclerosis). As the deposits slowly narrow your coronary arteries, your heart receives less blood. Eventually, diminished blood flow may cause chest pain (angina), shortness of breath or other symptoms. A complete blockage can cause a heart attack.

Since coronary artery disease often develops over decades, it can go virtually unnoticed until it produces a heart attack. But there's plenty you can do to prevent coronary artery disease. Start by committing to a healthy lifestyle.

Conventional Treatment

Lifestyle changes can promote healthier arteries. If you smoke, quitting is the most important thing you can do. Eat healthy foods, and exercise regularly. Sometimes medication or procedures to improve blood flow are recommended as well.

Medications

Various drugs can be used to treat coronary artery disease, including:

Cholesterol medications. Aggressively lowering your low-density lipoprotein (LDL or "bad") cholesterol can slow, stop or even reverse the buildup of fatty deposits in your arteries. Boosting your high-density lipoprotein (HDL or "good") cholesterol may help, too. Your doctor can choose from a range of cholesterol medications, including drugs known as statins and fibrates.

Aspirin. A daily aspirin or other blood thinner can reduce the tendency of your blood to clot, which may help prevent obstruction of your coronary arteries. If you've had a heart attack, aspirin can help prevent future attacks.

Beta blockers. These drugs slow your heart rate and decrease your blood pressure, which decreases your heart's demand for oxygen. If you've had a heart attack, beta blockers reduce the risk of future attacks.

Nitroglycerin. Nitroglycerin tablets, spray and patches can control chest pain by opening up your coronary arteries and reducing your heart's demand for blood.

Angiotensin-converting enzyme (ACE) inhibitors. These drugs decrease blood pressure and may help prevent progression of coronary artery disease. If you've had a heart attack, ACE inhibitors reduce the risk of future attacks.

Calcium channel blockers. These medications relax the muscles that surround your coronary arteries and cause the vessels to open, increasing blood flow to your heart. They also control high blood pressure.

Procedures to restore and improve blood flow

Sometimes more aggressive treatment is needed. On the next page are a few options.

Angioplasty and stent placement (percutaneous coronary revascularization). In this procedure, your doctor inserts a long, thin tube (catheter) into the narrowed part of your artery. A wire with a deflated balloon is passed through the catheter to the narrowed area. The balloon is then inflated, compressing the deposits against your artery walls. A mesh tube (stent) is often left in the artery to help keep the artery open. Some stents slowly release medication to help keep the artery open.

Coronary artery bypass surgery. A surgeon creates a graft to bypass blocked coronary arteries using a vessel from another part of your body. This allows blood to flow around the blocked or narrowed coronary artery. Because this requires open-heart surgery, it's most often reserved for cases of multiple narrowed coronary arteries.

Coronary brachytherapy. If the coronary arteries narrow again after stent placement, radiation may be used to help open the artery again.

Laser revascularization. If standard treatments aren't effective, a new surgery known as laser revascularization may be considered. During this procedure, a laser beam is used to make tiny new channels in the wall of the heart muscle. New vessels may grow through these channels and into the heart to provide additional paths for blood flow.

Complementary & Alternative Treatment

In relation to coronary artery disease, therapies focus primarily on reducing stress and lowering cholesterol (see page 149) or triglycerides.

Yoga. Yoga, with its emphasis on relaxation, fitness and a healthy lifestyle, may complement standard therapies for coronary artery disease. It may also improve heart disease risk factors such as high blood pressure, high cholesterol and high blood sugar levels. It's generally considered safe, but certain positions may pose a risk if you have spine problems, atherosclerosis of neck arteries, glaucoma or other medical problems. Check with your doctor before starting yoga if you have medical conditions.

Omega-3 fatty acids. There appears to be good evidence that omega-3 fatty acids (fish oil), from fish or from supplements, can reduce high triglyceride levels, which are a risk factor for coronary artery disease. Fish oil contains both docosahexaenoic acid (DHA) and eicosapentaenoic acid (EPA). Omega-3 fatty acids are also found in some plant and nut oils.

The American Heart Association recommends 2 to 4 grams (2,000 to 4,000 milligrams) of omega-3 fatty acids daily for people with elevated triglyceride levels. In addition, the association recommends 1 gram (1,000 mg) a day for people with documented coronary artery disease. The supplements should be taken in consultation with a doctor.

The effects of omega-3 supplements haven't been well studied beyond three months. Because high doses can cause bleeding, don't take more than 3 grams (3,000 mg) a day unless instructed to do so by your doctor.

Reducing your risk

Lifestyle changes can help you prevent or slow the progression of coronary artery disease.

- **Stop smoking.** Stopping is the best way to reduce your risk of a heart attack.
- **Control your blood pressure.** Have a blood pressure measurement at least every two years.
- **Check your cholesterol.** Have a baseline cholesterol test when you're in your 20s and then at least every five years.
- **Keep diabetes under control.** Blood sugar control can reduce the risk of heart disease.
- **Get moving.** Exercise helps you achieve and maintain a healthy weight and control diabetes, high cholesterol and high blood pressure — all coronary artery disease risk factors.
- **Eat healthy foods.** Focus on fruits, vegetables and whole grains.
- **Maintain a healthy weight.** Weight loss is especially important for people who have large waist measurements — more than 40 inches for men and more than 35 inches for women.
- **Manage stress.** Practice techniques for managing stress (see page 176).

The cholesterol connection

Cholesterol is found in every cell in your body. This fat-like substance is an important component of cell membranes and a building block in the formation of some hormones. But your body makes all the cholesterol it needs. Any cholesterol in your diet is extra — and it's up to no good.

When there's too much cholesterol in your blood, you may develop fatty deposits in your blood vessels. Eventually, these deposits make it difficult for enough blood to flow through your arteries. Your heart may not get as much oxygen-rich blood as it needs, which increases the risk of a heart attack. Decreased blood flow to your brain can cause a stroke.

But there's good news. High blood cholesterol (hypercholesterolemia) is largely preventable. A healthy diet, regular exercise and other lifestyle changes can go a long way toward reducing high cholesterol. Sometimes medication is needed, too.

Treating high cholesterol

Lifestyle changes play an important role and can help improve your cholesterol level. Eat a healthy diet, get regular physical activity and, if you smoke, stop. If you've made these important lifestyle changes and your total cholesterol — particularly your LDL cholesterol — remains high, your doctor may recommend medication.

Medications

The specific choice of medication or combination of medications depends on various factors, including your individual risk factors, your age, your current health and possible side effects. Common choices include:

- **Statins.** Statins — among the most commonly prescribed medications for lowering cholesterol — block a substance your liver needs to make cholesterol. This depletes cholesterol in your liver cells, which causes your liver to remove cholesterol from your blood. Statins may also help your body reabsorb cholesterol from accumulated deposits on your artery walls, potentially reversing coronary artery disease. Choices include atorvastatin (Lipitor), fluvastatin (Lescol), lovastatin (Altoprev, Mevacor), pravastatin (Pravachol), rosuvastatin (Crestor) and simvastatin (Zocor).

- **Bile-acid-binding resins.** Your liver uses cholesterol to make bile acids, a substance needed for digestion. The medications cholestyramine (Prevalite, Questran), colesevelam (WelChol) and colestipol (Colestid) lower cholesterol indirectly by binding to bile acids. This prompts your liver to use excess cholesterol to make more bile acids, which reduces the level of cholesterol in your blood.

- **Cholesterol absorption inhibitors.** Your small intestine absorbs the cholesterol from your diet and releases it into your bloodstream. The drug ezetimibe (Zetia) helps reduce blood cholesterol by limiting the absorption of dietary cholesterol. Zetia can be used in combination with any of the statin drugs.

- **Combination cholesterol absorption inhibitor and statin.** Ezetimibe-simvastatin (Vytorin) decreases both absorption of dietary cholesterol in your small intestine and production of cholesterol in your liver.

If you also have high triglycerides, your doctor may prescribe:

- **Fibrates.** The medications fenofibrate (Lofibra, TriCor) and gemfibrozil (Lopid) decrease triglycerides by reducing your liver's production of very-low-density lipoprotein (VLDL) cholesterol and by speeding up the removal of triglycerides from your blood. VLDL cholesterol contains mostly triglycerides.

- **Niacin.** Niacin (Niaspan) decreases triglycerides by limiting your liver's ability to produce LDL and VLDL cholesterol. Various prescription and non-prescription preparations are available, but prescription niacin is preferred. Dietary supplements containing niacin aren't effective for lowering triglycerides.

Most of these medications are well tolerated, but effectiveness varies from person to person. The most common side effects are stomach pain, constipation, nausea and diarrhea. If you decide to take cholesterol medication, your doctor may recommend periodic liver function tests to monitor the medication's effect on your liver.

Beyond the basics

In addition to standard medications, some complementary and alternative therapies may help lower cholesterol. Research suggests these therapies may offer benefits, and the risks appear to be relatively low.

- **Plant sterols or stanols.** These plant components help block the absorption of cholesterol and can lower LDL ("bad") cholesterol. They're now added to some foods, including margarines, orange juice and salad dressings. They're generally considered safe in recommended amounts, but caution should be used if you have certain medical conditions, including asthma or other respiratory conditions, diabetes or allergies to pine. Talk to your doctor. The American Heart Association recommends plant sterols or stanols only for people who have high levels of LDL cholesterol.

- **Psyllium.** Also called ispaghula, this comes from the husks of the seeds of *Plantago ovata* and is high in soluble dietary fiber. It's the main ingredient in many bulk laxatives and has some cholesterol-lowering effect. It's generally considered safe, except for people with significant bowel abnormalities or those who have had bowel surgery. In addition, people who frequently handle psyllium can be at risk of hypersensitivity reactions.

- **Beta-glucans.** This comes from a variety of sources, including plants, yeast, algae, bacteria and fungi. It's a soluble fiber, and as such, consumption is associated with a modest reduction in cholesterol. It's generally considered safe when taken orally.

- **Soy.** Long thought to have cholesterol-lowering effects, a recent meta-analysis by the American Heart Association's Nutrition Committee showed soy protein actually has very little impact on reducing cholesterol levels. In January 2006, the American Heart Association issued a statement saying the cardiovascular health benefits of soy protein are minimal at best. Although it may not lower your cholesterol, soy does contain vitamins and minerals and is a good source of fiber. It's also a healthy low-fat alternative source of protein.

- **Garlic.** Research indicates that garlic may lower cholesterol in the short term, but long-term results are unclear. The supplements appear to be of low risk, except in people taking anti-clotting medications.

Popular supplement policosanol may not reduce cholesterol

A new study reports that the popular nutritional supplement policosanol does not appear to reduce cholesterol levels, as previously thought.

Earlier studies suggested that policosanol reduced total cholesterol and low-density lipoprotein (LDL or "bad") cholesterol. Policosanol was also reported to boost high-density lipoprotein (HDL or "good") cholesterol. Most of these studies were supported by a single research group.

The latest study — which included 143 participants from multiple sites and a placebo control group — found no distinct link between policosanol and changes in cholesterol levels.

Because of the conflicting data, more definitive studies are needed.

Depression

Depression is a disorder that affects your thoughts, moods, feelings, behavior and even your physical health. People used to think it was "all in your head" and that if you really tried, you could "snap out of it" or just "get over it." But doctors now know that depression is not a weakness, and it's not something you can treat on your own. Depression is a medical disorder with a biological and chemical basis.

Sometimes, a stressful life event triggers depression. Other times, depression seems to occur spontaneously with no identifiable specific cause. Depression is much more than grieving or a bout of the blues.

Depression may occur only once in a person's life. Often, however, it occurs as repeated episodes over a lifetime, with periods free of depression in between. Or it may be a chronic condition, requiring ongoing treatment over a lifetime.

People of all ages and races are affected by depression. Medications are available that are generally safe and effective, even for the most severe depression. With proper treatment, most people with serious depression improve, often within weeks, and can return to normal daily activities.

Conventional Treatment

The development of newer antidepressant medications and mood-stabilizing drugs has improved the treatment of depression. Medications can relieve symptoms of depression and have become the first line of treatment for most types of the disorder.

Treatment may also include psychotherapy, which may help you cope with ongoing problems that may trigger or contribute to depression. A combination of medications and a brief course of psychotherapy usually is effective if you have mild to moderate depression. If you're severely depressed, initial treatment usually is with medications or electroconvulsive therapy. Once you improve, psychotherapy can be more effective.

Doctors usually treat depression in two stages. Acute treatment with medications helps relieve symptoms until you feel well. Once your symptoms ease, maintenance treatment typically continues for four to nine months to prevent a relapse. It's important to keep taking your medication even though you feel fine and are back to your usual activities. Episodes of depression recur in the majority of people who have one episode, but continuing treatment greatly reduces your risk of a rapid relapse. If you've had two or more previous episodes of depression, your doctor may suggest long-term treatment with antidepressants.

Medications

Selective serotonin reuptake inhibitors (SSRIs), such as fluoxetine (Prozac, Sarafem), paroxetine (Paxil), sertraline (Zoloft), citalopram (Celexa) and escitalopram (Lexapro), are often first-line treatments. Among tricyclic antidepressants are amitriptyline, desipramine (Norpramin), nortriptyline (Aventyl, Pamelor), protriptyline (Vivactil), trimipramine (Surmontil) and a combination of perphenazine and amitriptyline. Tetracyclics include maprotiline and mirtazapine (Remeron).

Other drugs include monoamine oxidase inhibitors (MAOIs), such as phenelzine (Nardil) and tranylcypromine (Parnate), and stimulants such as methylphenidate (Ritalin, Concerta), dextroamphetamine (Dexedrine, Dextrostat) or modafinil (Provigil). Doctors also prescribe lithium (Eskalith, Lithobid) and various mood-stabilizing drugs.

Psychotherapy

There are several types of psychotherapy. Each type involves a short-term, goal-oriented approach aimed at helping you deal with a specific issue. Prolonged psychotherapy is seldom necessary to treat depression.

Electroconvulsive therapy

Despite the images that many people conjure up, electroconvulsive therapy is generally safe and effective. Experts aren't sure how this therapy relieves the signs and symptoms of depression. The procedure may affect levels of neurotransmitters in your brain. The most common side effect is confusion that lasts a few minutes to several hours. This therapy is usually used for people who don't respond to medications and for those at high risk of suicide.

Light therapy

Light therapy may help if you have seasonal affective disorder. This disorder involves periods of depression that recur at the same time each year, usually when days are shorter in the fall and winter. Scientists believe fewer hours of sunlight may increase levels of melatonin, a brain hormone thought to induce sleep and depress mood. Treatment in the morning with a specialized type of bright light, which suppresses production of melatonin, may help if you have this disorder.

Complementary & Alternative Treatment

Some popular supplements marketed or taken for depression include:

St. John's wort. European studies suggest that St. John's wort may work as well as antidepressants in mild depression and with fewer side effects, but some studies have found that it isn't effective for major depression. Adverse reactions may include dry mouth, dizziness, digestive problems, fatigue, headache and sexual problems. In most cases, signs and symptoms are mild. St. John's wort can interfere with the effectiveness of prescription medications, including antidepressants, drugs to treat human immunodeficiency virus (HIV) infections and AIDS, and drugs to prevent organ rejection in people who've had transplants. If you take *any* prescription medication, talk to your doctor before taking St. John's wort.

SAM-e. This is a chemical substance found in all human cells and it plays a role in many body functions. It's thought to increase levels of serotonin and dopamine. Some studies have found SAM-e to be more effective than a placebo, but it's uncertain if it's as effective as conventional antidepressant medications. SAM-e can cause nausea and constipation.

5-HTP. One of the raw materials that your body needs to make serotonin is a chemical called 5-HTP, which is short for 5-hydroxytryptophan. In theory, if you boost your body's level of 5-HTP, you should also elevate your levels of serotonin. But there's not enough evidence to determine if 5-HTP is effective, and there are concerns about its safety.

Omega-3 fatty acids. Found in fish oil and certain nuts and plants, the acids are being studied as a possible mood stabilizer for people with bipolar depression and other psychiatric disorders.

Some nonsupplement therapies may help

Although supplements are popular for depression, a number of other integrative therapies may help. Work with your doctor to find how these may be used with conventional therapies.

Traditional Chinese medicine. This system, which broadly includes acupuncture, herbal remedies and massage, may provide some help for depression. For example, some studies suggest that acupuncture might be beneficial for depression. Overall, though, the research is inconclusive.

Art therapy. Self-expression through art therapy may help you deal with anxiety, stress, depression, and other mental and emotional issues.

Music therapy. Music therapy can enhance mood, promote relaxation and reduce anxiety.

Spirituality. Prayer may help you develop stronger coping skills and may reduce anxiety.

Electromagnetic therapy. Transcranial electromagnetic stimulation (TMS) is being studied at Mayo Clinic as a possible treatment for depression.

Yoga. As an exercise and as a meditative approach, yoga can enhance relaxation and help reduce anxiety.

Diabetes

Type 2 diabetes is a chronic condition that affects the way your body metabolizes sugar (glucose) — your body's main source of fuel.

Type 2 diabetes develops when your body becomes resistant to the effects of insulin — a hormone that regulates the absorption of sugar into your cells — or when your body produces some, but not enough, insulin to maintain a normal glucose level.

Nearly 21 million people in the United States have diabetes, according to the American Diabetes Association. About 90 percent to 95 percent of people with diabetes have type 2 diabetes. And the condition is on the rise, fueled largely by the current obesity epidemic.

The American Diabetes Association estimates that nearly one-third of people who have type 2 diabetes don't even know it. If the condition is left uncontrolled, the consequences can be life-threatening.

There's no cure for type 2 diabetes, but there's plenty you can do to manage — or prevent — the condition. Start by eating healthy foods, getting plenty of exercise and maintaining a healthy weight. If diet and exercise aren't enough, managing your blood sugar with medication can help you continue to live a healthy and active life.

Conventional Treatment

Eating a healthy diet, exercising and maintaining a healthy weight may be all that's needed to control your diabetes. When those aren't enough, you may need the help of medication.

Diet

Contrary to popular belief, there's no single diabetes diet. And having diabetes doesn't mean you have to eat only bland, boring foods. Instead, it means you'll eat more fruits, vegetables and whole grains and fewer animal products and sweets. It's the same eating plan that's recommended for everyone. A registered dietitian can help you create a meal plan that fits your health goals, food preferences and lifestyle. To keep your blood sugar consistent, try to eat the same amount of food with the same proportion of carbohydrates, proteins and fats at the same time every day.

Exercise

The same exercises that are good for your heart and lungs also help lower your blood sugar levels. Consult your doctor before beginning an exercise program.

Maintaining a healthy weight

Fat makes your cells more resistant to insulin. But when you lose weight, the process reverses and your cells become more receptive to insulin. For some people with type 2 diabetes, weight loss is all that's needed to restore blood sugar to normal.

Medication

Various drugs may be used to treat type 2 diabetes, including:

Sulfonylurea drugs. These medications stimulate your pancreas to produce and release more insulin, as long as your pancreas already produces some insulin on its own. Second-generation sulfonylureas such as glipizide (Glucotrol, Glucotrol XL), glyburide (DiaBeta, Glynase, Micronase) and glimepiride (Amaryl) are prescribed most often.

Meglitinides. These medications, such as repaglinide (Prandin), have effects similar to sulfonylureas, but they're not as likely to lead to low blood sugar. Meglitinides work quickly, and the results fade rapidly.

Biguanides. Metformin (Glucophage, Glucophage XR) is the only drug in this class available in the United States. It works by inhibiting the production and release of glucose from your liver, which means you need less insulin to transport blood sugar into your cells.

Alpha-glucosidase inhibitors. These drugs block the action of enzymes in your digestive tract that break down carbohydrates. This means sugar is absorbed into your bloodstream more slowly, which helps prevent the rapid rise in blood sugar that usually occurs right after a meal. Drugs in this class include acarbose (Precose) and miglitol (Glyset).

Thiazolidinediones. These drugs, such as rosiglitazone (Avandia) and pioglitazone hydrochloride (Actos), make your body tissues more sensitive to insulin and keep your liver from overproducing glucose.

Insulin. Some people with type 2 diabetes must take insulin every day to replace what their pancreas is unable to produce.

Amylin mimetics. The first in this new class of drugs, pramlintide (Symlin), mimics the action of amylin, a protein secreted by the pancreas. This medication slows down the movement of food through your stomach after meals, affecting how rapidly glucose enters your bloodstream.

Incretin mimetics. First in another new class of drugs, exenatide (Byetta) mimics the action of the hormone incretin, which helps regulate fasting glucose levels and glucose levels after meals.

Complementary & Alternative Treatment

Several therapies may have some benefit for diabetes and appear to be low risk. Work with your doctor when considering these, as you will need to monitor your blood sugar carefully, and you may need to modify the dose of your conventional medication to avoid low blood sugar.

Bitter melon. Research — including research on safety — is limited, but this herb appears to lower blood sugar. It should not be used by children or pregnant women.

Cinnamon. Cinnamon taken orally appears to lower blood sugar, possibly by making the body more sensitive to insulin. It's likely safe when taken in amounts commonly found in foods, and may be safe in recommended doses in supplement form.

Ginseng. This herb is used widely for a number of conditions, including diabetes, and appears to have little risk of serious side effects when taken in recommended doses.

Gymnema. Leaves of this plant have been used for centuries in India to treat diabetes, and research has not identified negative side effects.

Stevia. Stevia (*Stevia rebaudiana*) is a traditional South American treatment for diabetes, and it's used as a sweetener in Brazil and Japan. It should not be confused with *Stevia salicifolia*, which is also called ronion.

Not recommended

Fenugreek. Potential risks, such as a possible increased risk of bleeding, outweigh the unproven benefits for diabetes of this herb.

Other therapies to control blood sugar

Several small studies indicate that **yoga** may help in the treatment of diabetes. Studies conducted in India found a decrease in blood sugar following yoga sessions. One study suggested that the result was due to the effects of yoga on the pancreas. Yoga is considered a relatively low-risk integrative therapy.

Another traditional Indian practice, **ayurveda,** is also used for diabetes, but study results are mixed. Ayurveda involves the use of, among other things, herbs, massage, diet and exercise to cleanse the body and restore energy balance. Some studies have shown modest benefits for diabetes, but the practice has not been well-researched. In addition, there are concerns that some ayurvedic medications could be toxic. If you try ayurvedic practices, do so with caution.

Traditional Chinese medicine also may have some benefits for managing diabetes. Acupuncture, which is part of traditional Chinese medicine, has been shown to reduce pain associated with diabetic neuropathy. However, there may be significant risks from unproven Chinese herbs and herb combinations if you ignore conventional therapies, or if don't continue to monitor your blood sugar closely.

Fibromyalgia

You hurt all over and frequently feel exhausted. Even after numerous tests, your doctor can't seem to find anything specifically wrong with you. If this sounds familiar, you may have fibromyalgia.

Fibromyalgia is a chronic condition characterized by fatigue, widespread pain in your muscles, ligaments and tendons, and multiple tender points — places on your body where slight pressure causes pain. Fibromyalgia is more common in women than in men. Previously, the condition was known by other names such as fibrositis, chronic muscle pain syndrome, psychogenic rheumatism and tension myalgias.

Although the intensity of symptoms may vary, they typically never disappear completely. It may be reassuring to know, however, that fibromyalgia isn't progressive, crippling or life-threatening. Treatments and self-care steps can improve symptoms and your general health.

Conventional Treatment

In general, treatment for fibromyalgia involves a combination of medication and self-care. The emphasis is on minimizing symptoms and improving general health.

Medications
Medications can help reduce the pain of fibromyalgia and improve sleep. Common choices include:

Analgesics. Acetaminophen (Tylenol, others) may ease the pain and stiffness caused by fibromyalgia. However, its effectiveness varies. Tramadol (Ultram) is a prescription pain reliever that may be taken with or without acetaminophen. Your doctor may recommend nonsteroidal anti-inflammatory drugs (NSAIDs) — such as aspirin, ibuprofen (Advil, Motrin, others) or naproxen sodium (Anaprox, Aleve) — in conjunction with other medications, but NSAIDs haven't proved to be effective in managing the pain of fibromyalgia when taken by themselves.

Antidepressants. Your doctor may prescribe antidepressant medications, such as amitriptyline, nortriptyline (Aventyl, Pamelor) or doxepin (Sinequan) to help promote sleep. Fluoxetine (Prozac) in combination with amitriptyline has also been found effective. Sertraline (Zoloft) and paroxetine (Paxil) can help if you're experiencing depression.

Muscle relaxants. Taking the medication cyclobenzaprine (Flexeril) at bedtime may help treat muscle pain and spasms. Muscle relaxants are generally limited to short-term use.

Other medications. Prescription sleeping pills, such as zolpidem (Ambien), may provide short-term benefits for some people with fibromyalgia, but doctors usually advise against long-term use of these drugs. These medications tend to work for only a short time, after which your body becomes resistant to their effects. Ultimately, using sleeping pills tends to create even more sleeping problems in many people.

Benzodiazepines may help relax muscles and promote sleep, but doctors often avoid these drugs in treating fibromyalgia. Benzodiazepines can become habit-forming, and they haven't provided long-term benefits.

Doctors don't usually recommend narcotics for treating fibromyalgia because of the potential for dependence and addiction. Corticosteroids, such as prednisone, haven't been shown to be effective in treating fibromyalgia.

Cognitive behavior therapy
Cognitive behavior therapy seeks to increase your belief in your own abilities and teaches you methods for dealing with stressful situations. Therapy can be provided via individual counseling, audiotapes or classes, and may help you manage your fibromyalgia.

Treatment programs

Interdisciplinary treatment programs may be effective in improving your symptoms, including relieving pain. These programs can combine a variety of treatments, such as relaxation techniques, biofeedback, and gentle, graded exercise. Receiving information and learning about chronic pain can be very helpful. There isn't one combination that works best for everybody. Your doctor can create a program based on what works best for you.

Complementary & Alternative Treatment

Several integrative treatments do appear to safely relieve stress and reduce pain, but many practices remain unproved because they haven't been adequately studied. Commonly used therapies include:

Acupuncture. Results of a Mayo Clinic study released in June 2006 showed that symptoms among fibromyalgia participants who received acupuncture significantly improved compared with a control group. The study involved 50 individuals enrolled in a randomized, controlled trial. Acupuncture is generally a low-risk treatment. Make sure to find an experienced practitioner.

Massage. This is a relatively safe way to relax tense muscles and help ease pain.

Relaxation therapy. A broad range of therapies, from guided imagery to meditation and progressive muscle relaxation, fall under this heading. These are low-risk techniques that may have some benefits.

5-HTP. Limited research suggests some benefits, such as reducing the number of tender points, improving sleep and lessening anxiety, from this precursor for the brain chemical serotonin. But safety is uncertain and it should be used only with the supervision of a doctor.

Healing (therapeutic) touch. There's some limited evidence to show that this therapy, which seeks to manipulate energy fields around the body, may improve symptoms of fibromyalgia. There are few risks, aside from cost.

Use caution

SAM-e. Although this synthetic version of a substance naturally found in the body is used for fibromyalgia, two randomized, controlled studies found that it didn't have clinically significant benefits over an inactive pill (placebo) for fibromyalgia-related depression or for reducing tender points. Side effects can include flatulence, vomiting, diarrhea, headache and nausea. SAM-e can negatively interact with antidepressant medications.

DHEA. The steroid may be effective in treating mild depression, which can be associated with fibromyalgia, but long term use and high levels of the steroid may put you at risk of serious side effects.

Self-care for fibromyalgia

Self-care is critical in the management of fibromyalgia.

- **Reduce stress.** Develop a plan to avoid or limit overexertion and emotional stress. Allow yourself time each day to relax. But don't change your routine totally. People who quit work or drop all activity tend to do worse than those who remain active. Try stress management techniques, such as deep-breathing exercises or meditation.

- **Get enough sleep.** Because fatigue is one of the main characteristics of fibromyalgia, getting sufficient sleep is essential. In addition, practice good sleep habits, such as going to bed and getting up at the same time each day and limiting daytime napping.

- **Exercise regularly.** At first, exercise may increase your pain. But doing it regularly often decreases symptoms. Appropriate exercises often include walking, biking, swimming and water aerobics. A physical therapist can help you develop a home exercise program. Stretching, good posture and relaxation exercises also are helpful.

- **Pace yourself.** Keep your activity on an even level. If you do too much on your good days, you may have more bad days.

Hay fever

If spring brings a stuffy nose, scratchy eyes and an extra sneeze tacked on to your usual "achoo!" — you're likely very familiar with hay fever (allergic rhinitis).

Hay fever is the common name for an allergic response to specific substances in your environment. It's one of the most common allergic reactions, affecting about 40 million people in the United States.

If you have seasonal hay fever, tree pollen, grasses or weeds may trigger your symptoms. If you're sensitive to indoor allergens such as dust mites, cockroaches, mold or pet dander, you may have year-round symptoms.

Nonprescription medications and self-care measures may be enough to manage your mild hay fever symptoms. But if your signs and symptoms are more severe — or if hay fever is a year-round nuisance — see an allergy specialist for evaluation and treatment.

Without proper treatment, hay fever can cause sleeplessness, fatigue and irritability, possibly affecting your performance at work or school. It can also increase your risk of developing more serious allergic conditions such as asthma or eczema.

Conventional Treatment

Typically, the first step in dealing with hay fever is identifying what triggers your symptoms, then helping you develop a plan to avoid these substances. In some cases, avoidance alone can effectively control hay fever problems. Your doctor may also prescribe an oral medication, a nasal spray or eyedrops — alone or in combination — to decrease your signs and symptoms. Conventional treatments for hay fever include:

Medications

Nasal corticosteroids. These are the most effective hay fever medications and are often prescribed first, especially for more troublesome signs and symptoms. Examples include beclomethasone (Beconase) and fluticasone propionate (Flonase). They're generally safe for extended use. Mild side effects can include an unpleasant smell or taste and nasal irritation.

Antihistamines. These oral medications and nasal sprays help relieve itching, sneezing and runny nose but have less effect on congestion. Nonprescription oral antihistamines include diphenhydramine (Benadryl) and chlorpheniramine (Chlor-Trimeton), while prescription drugs include cetirizine (Zyrtec) and fexofenadine (Allegra). Some can cause drowsiness.

Decongestants. Often used in combination with antihistamines, these are available in nonprescription and prescription liquids, tablets and nasal sprays. Oral decongestants include pseudoephedrine (Sudafed, Actifed, others). Nasal decongestants include phenylephrine (Neo-Synephrine) and oxymetazoline (Afrin). Avoid them if you have high blood pressure (hypertension). Oral decongestants can worsen the symptoms of prostate enlargement, making urination more difficult.

Cromolyn sodium. This nonprescription nasal spray (NasalCrom, others) helps relieve hay fever symptoms by preventing the release of histamine. It's not associated with any serious side effects.

Leukotriene modifier. Montelukast (Singulair) is a prescription tablet that blocks leukotrienes — immune system chemicals that cause allergy symptoms such as excess mucus production. Possible side effects include headache and, less commonly, abdominal pain, cough and dental pain.

Nasal atropine. Available in a prescription nasal spray, ipratropium bromide (Atrovent) helps relieve a severe runny nose by preventing the glands in your nose from producing excess fluid. Mild side effects include nasal dryness, nosebleeds and sore throat. Rarely, it can cause more severe side effects such as blurred vision, dizziness and difficult urination. It's not recommended if you have glaucoma or an enlarged prostate.

If you're taking any other medications or have a chronic health condition, talk to your doctor or pharmacist before starting any treatment for hay fever, to be sure you're not at risk of a drug interaction or other adverse effect.

Allergy shots

If medications don't relieve your symptoms, your doctor may recommend allergy shots (immunotherapy or desensitization therapy). Over three to five years, you receive injections containing purified allergen extracts. The goal is to desensitize you to specific allergens.

Self-care

For pollen and molds. Close doors and windows during pollen season. Use air conditioning in your house and car. Stay indoors on dry, windy days. Use a high-efficiency particulate air (HEPA) filter in your bedroom.

For dust mites. Use allergy-proof covers on mattresses and pillows. Wash sheets and blankets in at least 130 F water. Vacuum carpets weekly with a small-particle or HEPA filter. Consider removing carpet.

For pet dander. Remove pets from the house and bathe pets weekly. If pets are in the house, keep them out of your bedroom.

Complementary & Alternative Treatment

Nasal irrigation and butterbur are two common alternative therapies for hay fever. Of the two, irrigation seems to have more benefit and less risk.

Common therapies

Nasal irrigation. This therapy is often associated with yoga. There are several variations, but one common technique uses a small container, called a neti pot, that you fill with a mild solution of warm salt water. You tip your head forward and slightly sideways over a sink and place the tip of the pot's spout in one nostril. The solution runs in that nostril, through your sinuses and out the other nostril. Repeat on the other side.

The therapy appears to have little risk and is recommended by the International Consensus Report on the Diagnosis and Treatment of Rhinitis. If you have frequent nosebleeds, have had recent nose surgery, or your gag reflex is impaired, talk with your doctor before trying this.

Butterbur. Extracts of this shrub may have some effectiveness in preventing hay fever symptoms. But, because raw butterbur contains potentially toxic substances, use only a commercially prepared product labeled PA-free. Safety of use in children and use beyond 12 to 16 weeks are unknown. Don't take with other medications without doctor supervision.

Other therapies. Probiotics, acupuncture, aromatherapy and hypnosis are also used for hay fever. Benefits are uncertain but risks appear low.

Conflicting or unclear evidence

Other therapies, including cat's claw, choline, goldenseal, stinging nettle, belladonna and bromelain, have been promoted for hay fever, but the research is conflicting or not strong enough to recommend them.

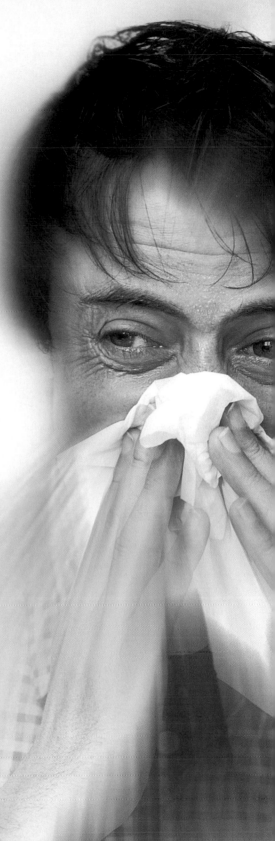

Headache

Although headache pain sometimes can be severe, in most cases it's not the result of an underlying disease. The vast majority of headaches are so-called primary headaches. These include migraine and tension headache.

A tension headache is the most common headache, and yet it's not well understood. A tension headache generally produces a diffuse, usually mild to moderate pain over your head. Many people liken the feeling to having a tight band around their head. In many cases, there's no clear cause for a tension headache.

Migraines affect more than 28 million Americans — three times more women than men. A migraine is often disabling. In some cases, these painful headaches are preceded or accompanied by a sensory warning sign (aura), such as flashes of light, blind spots or tingling in your arm or leg. A migraine can also often be accompanied by other signs and symptoms, such as nausea, vomiting, and extreme sensitivity to light and sound.

Managing headaches is often a balance between fostering healthy habits, finding effective nondrug treatments and using medications appropriately. In addition, a number of preventive, self-care and alternative treatments may help you deal with headache pain.

Conventional Treatment

Treatment for headaches depends on the type. Here's an overview of treatment options for two main types of headaches:

Tension headaches

A variety of medications, both nonprescription and prescription, are available for treating tension headaches. You may find fast, effective relief by taking pain relievers such as aspirin, ibuprofen (Advil, Motrin, others) or acetaminophen (Tylenol, others). These medications are inexpensive and readily available and don't require a prescription from your doctor. People with severe or chronic tension headache may require stronger painkillers or preventive medications. Which drug works best varies from one person to another.

Whether you have episodic or chronic headaches, don't overuse nonprescription medications. Limit your use of painkillers to two days a week. Try to take the medications only when necessary, and use the smallest dose needed to relieve your pain. Overusing pain medications can cause rebound headaches or the development of chronic daily headache, triggering the very symptoms you're trying to stop. In addition, all medications used to treat headache have side effects, some of which may be serious. For prescription medications, follow the recommended dosage.

Medications don't cure headaches, and over time painkillers and other medications may lose their effectiveness. If you take medications regularly, discuss the risks and benefits with your doctor. Also, remember that pain medications aren't a substitute for recognizing and dealing with the stressors that may be causing your headaches.

Migraines

Pain-relieving medications. These drugs are taken to stop pain once it has started. For best results, take pain-relieving drugs as soon as you experience signs or symptoms of a migraine. It may help if you rest or sleep in a dark room after taking them.

Examples include nonsteroidal anti-inflammatory drugs (NSAIDs), such as ibuprofen (Advil, Motrin, others) or aspirin, triptans, such as sumatriptan (Imitrex), rizatriptan (Maxalt) and naratriptan (Amerge), and ergots, such as ergotamine (Ergomar) and dihydroergotamine (D.H.E. 45).

Preventive medications. These drugs help reduce or prevent migraines. Choosing a preventive strategy depends on the frequency and severity of your headaches, the degree of disability your headaches cause and other medical conditions you may have. You may be a candidate for preventive therapy if you have two or more debilitating attacks a month, if you use pain-relieving medications more than twice a week, if pain-relieving medications aren't helping or if you have uncommon migraines.

Preventive medications include cardiovascular drugs such as beta blockers, calcium channel blockers — especially verapamil (Calan, Isoptin) — and the high blood pressure drugs lisinopril (Prinivil, Zestril) and candesartan (Atacand). Antidepressants — especially tricyclic antidepressants, such as amitriptyline, nortriptyline (Pamelor) and protriptyline (Vivactil) — are also used, as are NSAIDs and anti-seizure drugs such as divalproex sodium (Depakote), valproic acid (Depakene) and topiramate (Topamax).

Also on the list of preventive medications are cyproheptadine, an antihistamine that affects serotonin activity, and botulinum toxin type A (Botox), which is injected into the muscles of the face and head.

Complementary & Alternative Treatment

Nontraditional therapies used for headache pain include:

Acupuncture. Among other benefits, acupuncture may be helpful for headache pain. This treatment uses thin, disposable needles that generally cause little or no pain or discomfort. Find an experienced practitioner.

Biofeedback. Biofeedback appears to be effective in relieving migraine pain. This relaxation technique uses special equipment to teach you how to monitor and control certain physical responses, such as muscle tension.

Massage. Although massage is a wonderful way to reduce stress and relieve tension, its value in treating headaches hasn't been fully determined. For people who have tight, tender muscles in the back of the head, neck and shoulders, massage may help relieve headache pain.

Herbs, vitamins and minerals. There is some evidence that the herbs feverfew and butterbur may prevent migraines or reduce their severity. A high dose of riboflavin (vitamin B-2) also may prevent migraines by correcting tiny deficiencies in the brain cells. Magnesium supplements may reduce the frequency of headaches in some people, although studies don't all agree on this issue. In addition, infusions of magnesium sulfate seem to help some people during an acute headache, and they seem to relieve migraine pain in people with magnesium deficiencies. Ask your doctor if these treatments are right for you. Don't use feverfew or butterbur if you're pregnant.

Use caution

Although some people use hypnosis and the supplement 5-HTP for headaches, there's limited evidence that these are effective.

High blood pressure

You can have high blood pressure (hypertension) for years without a single symptom. But silence isn't golden in this case. Uncontrolled high blood pressure increases your risk of serious health problems, including heart attack and stroke.

Blood pressure is determined by the amount of blood your heart pumps and the amount of resistance to blood flow in your arteries. The more blood your heart pumps and the narrower your arteries, the higher your blood pressure.

High blood pressure typically develops without signs or symptoms. It affects nearly a third of Americans adults, and about half of Americans age 60 and older, according to the National Heart, Lung, and Blood Institute. Fortunately, high blood pressure can be easily detected. And once you know you have high blood pressure, you can work with your doctor to control it.

Conventional Treatment

Changing your lifestyle can go a long way toward controlling high blood pressure. But sometimes lifestyle changes aren't enough. In addition to diet and exercise, your doctor may recommend medication.

Which category of medication your doctor prescribes depends on your stage of high blood pressure and whether you also have other medical conditions. To reduce the number of doses you need a day, which can reduce side effects, your doctor may prescribe a combination of low-dose medications rather than larger doses of one single drug. In fact, two or more blood pressure drugs often work better than one.

The major types of medication used for high blood pressure include:

Thiazide diuretics. These medications act on your kidneys to help your body eliminate sodium and water, reducing blood volume. Thiazide diuretics are often the first — but not the only — choice in high blood pressure medications. In a 2006 study, diuretics were a key factor in preventing heart failure associated with high blood pressure.

Beta blockers. These medications reduce the workload on your heart, causing your heart to beat slower and with less force. When prescribed alone, beta blockers don't work as well in blacks — but they're effective when combined with a thiazide diuretic.

Angiotensin-converting enzyme (ACE) inhibitors. These medications help relax blood vessels by blocking the formation of a natural chemical that narrows blood vessels. ACE inhibitors may be especially important in treating high blood pressure in people with coronary artery disease, heart failure or kidney failure. Like beta blockers, ACE inhibitors don't work as well in blacks when prescribed alone, but they're effective when combined with a thiazide diuretic.

Angiotensin II receptor blockers. These medications help relax blood vessels by blocking the action — not the formation — of a natural chemical that narrows blood vessels. Like ACE inhibitors, angiotensin II receptor blockers often are useful for people with coronary artery disease, heart failure and kidney failure.

Calcium channel blockers. These medications help relax the muscles of your blood vessels. Some slow your heart rate. A word of caution for grapefruit lovers. Grapefruit juice interacts with some calcium channel blockers, increasing blood levels of the medication and putting you at higher risk of side effects. Researchers have identified the substance in grapefruit juice that causes the interaction, which may one day lead to commercial grapefruit juices that don't pose such a risk.

If you're having trouble reaching your blood pressure goal with combinations of the above medications, your doctor may prescribe:

Alpha blockers. These medications reduce nerve impulses to blood vessels, reducing the effects of natural chemicals that narrow vessels.

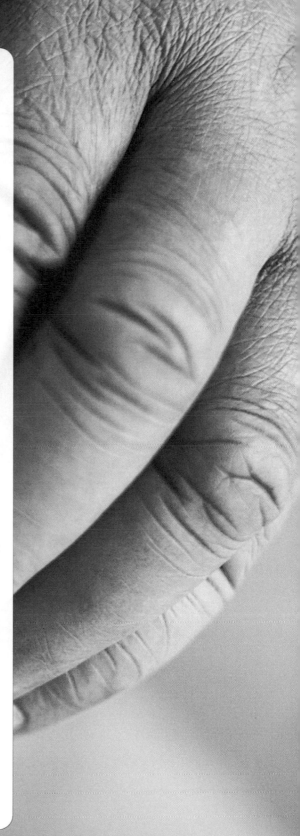

Alpha-beta blockers. In addition to reducing nerve impulses to blood vessels, alpha-beta blockers slow the heartbeat to reduce the amount of blood that must be pumped through the vessels.

Central-acting agents. These prevent your brain from telling your nervous system to increase your heart rate and narrow your blood vessels.

Vasodilators. These medications work directly on the muscles in the walls of your arteries, preventing your arteries from narrowing.

Complementary & Alternative Treatment

Several integrative therapies appear to have value for high blood pressure.

Omega-3 fatty acids. Omega-3s can be found in fish oil and in some plant and nut oils. They have been found to lower blood pressure as well as triglycerides. However, doses may need to be higher than 3 grams (3,000 milligrams) a day to be effective, and amounts above 3 grams may increase the risk of bleeding, so work with your doctor.

Coenzyme Q10. Small decreases in blood pressure have been noted in research on coenzyme Q10, also called CoQ10. Side effects appear to be few at recommended doses, but long-term safety at higher doses is unknown. CoQ10 may lower blood sugar levels, so use it with caution if you're taking diabetes medications. In addition, vigorous exercise may cause negative side effects if you're using CoQ10 supplements.

Yoga. Yoga may improve high blood pressure, as well as high cholesterol and high blood sugar levels. It's generally considered safe, but certain positions may pose a risk if you have spine problems, atherosclerosis of neck arteries, glaucoma or other medical problems. Check with your doctor before starting yoga if you have serious or unstable medical conditions.

Qi gong. In combination with conventional therapies, this traditional Chinese practice may help lower blood pressure. There are many different forms of qi gong, ranging from a practitioner who uses his or her hands on a patient to forms that use meditation and exercise.

Paced respiration. Paced respiration refers to slow, deep breathing. In various clinical trials, regular use of an over-the-counter device that analyzes breathing patterns and helps guide inhalation and exhalation was found to help lower blood pressure. You can also practice such breathing on your own, without the use of a device.

Acupuncture. This traditional Chinese therapy involves the insertion of fine needles into the skin at certain points to restore proper energy flow. There's mixed evidence on its effectiveness for high blood pressure, but it's generally a low-risk treatment. Find an experienced practitioner.

Garlic. Garlic also falls into the mixed-evidence-but-low-risk category when it comes to high blood pressure. Amounts found in supplements are generally considered safe, unless you take anti-clotting medications. Work with your doctor.

Insomnia

Almost everyone has occasional sleepless nights, perhaps due to stress, heartburn, or drinking too much caffeine or alcohol. Insomnia is a lack of sleep that occurs on a regular or frequent basis, and often for no apparent reason.

How much sleep is enough varies from person to person. Although 7 ½ hours of sleep is about average, some people do well on four to five hours of sleep. Other people need nine to 10 hours of sleep each night.

Insomnia can affect not only your energy level and mood, but also your health because sleep helps bolster your immune system. Fatigue, at any age, leads to diminished mental alertness and concentration. Lack of sleep caused by insomnia is linked to accidents both on the road and on the job.

Insomnia may be either temporary or chronic. You don't necessarily have to live with the sleepless nights of insomnia. Some simple changes in your daily routine and habits may result in better sleep.

Conventional Treatment

No matter what your age, insomnia usually is treatable. The key often lies in changes to your routine during the day and when you go to bed.

Coping skills

Key coping skills that can help overcome sleep problems include:
- Sticking to a sleep schedule
- Limiting your time in bed
- Avoiding "trying" to sleep
- Hiding the bedroom clocks
- Exercising and staying active
- Avoiding or limiting caffeine, alcohol and nicotine
- Checking your medications for drugs that may affect sleep
- Dealing with painful health conditions
- Finding ways to relax
- Avoiding or limiting naps
- Minimizing sleep interruptions

Medication

If self-help measures don't work or you believe that another condition, such as depression, restless legs syndrome or anxiety, is causing your insomnia, talk to your doctor. He or she may recommend that you take medications to promote relaxation or sleep.

Prescription medications. Taking prescription sleeping pills, such as zolpidem (Ambien), eszopiclone (Lunesta), zaleplon (Sonata) or ramelteon (Rozerem), for a couple of weeks until there's less stress in your life may help you get to sleep until you notice benefits from behavioral self-help measures. The antidepressant trazodone (Desyrel) also may help with insomnia.

Doctors generally don't recommend prescription sleeping pills for the long term because they may cause side effects. Plus, your goal is to develop the ability to sleep without the help of medication. In addition, sleeping pills can become less effective after a while.

Nonprescription medications. Nonprescription sleep aids contain antihistamines to induce drowsiness. They're OK for occasional sleepless nights, but they, too, often lose their effectiveness the more you take them. Many sleeping pills contain diphenhydramine, which can cause difficulty urinating and a drowsy feeling in the daytime.

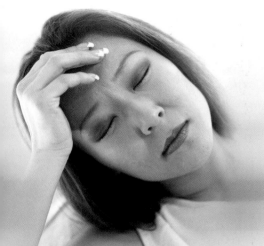

Complementary & Alternative Treatment

There are many nonconventional treatments used for insomnia, and several show promise.

Melatonin. Melatonin is a hormone produced naturally in the brain. Supplements contain synthetic melatonin. Although widely used for prevention of jet lag, it's also used for sleep problems, where it seems most effective in older people. Melatonin is generally considered safe at recommended levels but may cause clotting abnormalities in people taking the blood thinner warfarin (Coumadin). It shouldn't be taken if you're pregnant or trying to become pregnant.

Valerian. Research suggests that valerian, a perennial plant, may help you get to sleep faster and improve sleep quality. It's generally considered safe at recommended doses. It's also used for anxiety. Research from a multicenter study also suggests that the combination of valerian and hops may help insomnia.

Guided imagery. This can refer to a number of therapies, including visualization. The goal is to help you relax and visualize a positive outcome, in the case of insomnia, sleep. Guided imagery has been shown to alter breathing, heart rate and blood pressure. It's generally considered safe.

May help and likely won't hurt

Although research is unclear about the value of these therapies for insomnia, the risk of trying them is relatively low:

Acupuncture. A small Korean study of people 65 and older found acupuncture to be effective for insomnia, and another study found acupuncture helped insomnia during pregnancy.

Hypnosis. One study of school-age children found hypnosis beneficial in overcoming insomnia.

Lavender. A study of female college students found that lavender fragrance was effective for both insomnia and depression.

Music therapy. A small study of women in two domestic abuse centers found that music therapy improved sleep quality and also reduced anxiety.

Don't ignore sleep problems

Sleep is as important to your health as a healthy diet and regular exercise. Whatever your reason for sleep loss, insomnia can impact you both mentally and physically.

The impact can be cumulative. People with chronic insomnia are more likely than others to develop psychiatric problems such as depression and anxiety disorders. Long-term sleep deprivation can also increase the severity of chronic diseases, such as high blood pressure and diabetes.

And it's clear that insufficient sleep can lead to serious or even fatal accidents. According to the National Highway Traffic Safety Administration, more than 100,000 crashes each year are due to drivers falling asleep at the wheel.

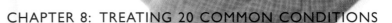

Irritable bowel syndrome

Irritable bowel syndrome (IBS) is one of the most common disorders that doctors see. Yet it's also one that many people aren't comfortable talking about.

Irritable bowel syndrome is characterized by abdominal pain or cramping and changes in bowel function — including bloating, gas, diarrhea and constipation — problems most people don't like to discuss. What's more, for many years irritable bowel syndrome was considered a psychological rather than a physical problem.

Up to one in five American adults has irritable bowel syndrome. The disorder accounts for more than one out of every 10 doctor visits. For most people, signs and symptoms of irritable bowel disease are mild. Only a small percentage of people have severe signs and symptoms.

Fortunately, unlike more serious intestinal diseases such as ulcerative colitis and Crohn's disease, irritable bowel syndrome doesn't cause inflammation or changes in bowel tissue or increase your risk of colorectal cancer. In many cases, you can control irritable bowel syndrome by managing your diet, lifestyle and stress.

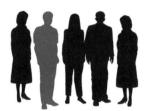

Up to one in five American adults has irritable bowel syndrome.

Conventional Treatment

Because it's still not clear what causes irritable bowel syndrome, treatment focuses on the relief of symptoms so that you can live your life as fully and normally as possible.

In most cases, you can successfully control mild symptoms of irritable bowel syndrome by learning to manage stress and making changes in your diet and lifestyle. But if your problems are moderate or severe, you may need more help than lifestyle changes alone can offer. Your doctor may suggest:

Fiber supplements. Taking fiber supplements such as psyllium (Metamucil) or methylcellulose (Citrucel) with fluids may help control constipation.

Anti-diarrheal medications. Over-the-counter medications such as loperamide (Imodium) can help control diarrhea.

Eliminating high-gas foods. If you have significant bloating or are passing significant amounts of gas, your doctor may also ask you to cut out such items as carbonated beverages, salads, raw fruits and vegetables, cabbage, broccoli and cauliflower.

Anticholinergic medications. Some people need drugs that affect certain activities of the nervous system (anticholinergics) to relieve painful bowel spasms.

Antidepressant medications. If your symptoms include pain and depression, your doctor may recommend a tricyclic antidepressant or a selective serotonin reuptake inhibitor (SSRI). These medications help relieve depression as well as inhibit the activity of neurons that control the intestines. For diarrhea and abdominal pain, your doctor may suggest tricyclic antidepressants, such as imipramine (Tofranil) and amitriptyline. Side effects of these drugs include drowsiness and constipation. SSRIs such as fluoxetine (Prozac, Sarafem) or paroxetine (Paxil) may be helpful if you're depressed and have pain and constipation.

Counseling. If antidepressant medications don't work, you may have better results from counseling if stress tends to exacerbate your symptoms.

Medications specifically for IBS

There are currently two drugs available to treat IBS: alosetron (Lotronex) and tegaserod (Zelnorm).

Alosetron. This drug is a nerve receptor antagonist that's supposed to relax the colon and slow the movement of waste through the lower bowel. But the drug was removed from the market just nine months after its approval when it was linked to at least four deaths and severe side effects in 197 people. In June 2002, the Food and Drug Administration (FDA) decided to allow alosetron to be sold again — with restrictions.

The drug can be prescribed only by doctors enrolled in a special program and is intended for severe cases of diarrhea-predominant IBS in women who don't respond to other treatments. It isn't approved for men.

Tegaserod. For women who have IBS with constipation, the FDA has approved the medication tegaserod (Zelnorm). It's approved for short-term use in women and hasn't been shown to be effective for treating men with IBS. Tegaserod imitates the action of the neurotransmitter serotonin and helps to coordinate the nerves and muscles in the intestine. Some reports have suggested a risk of rare, dangerous side effects similar to those of alosetron, but the drug is still available.

Complementary & Alternative Treatment

The following nontraditional therapies may help relieve symptoms of irritable bowel syndrome:

Probiotics. Probiotics are "good" bacteria that normally live in your intestines and are found in certain foods, such as yogurt, and in dietary supplements. It's been suggested that people with irritable bowel syndrome may not have enough good bacteria, and that adding probiotics to your diet may help ease your symptoms. Some studies have shown that probiotics can help IBS. Not all studies on probiotics have had positive results, however. Use of probiotics is generally considered safe at recommended doses.

Peppermint. Peppermint is a natural antispasmodic that relaxes smooth muscles in the intestines. Study results haven't been consistently encouraging, but if you'd like to try peppermint be sure to use enteric-coated capsules. Peppermint may aggravate heartburn. Before taking any herbs, check with your doctor to be sure they won't interact or interfere with other medications you may be taking.

Acupuncture. Researchers at the National Institutes of Health (NIH) have found that acupuncture can provide relief from chronic pain. Although study results on the effects of acupuncture on symptoms of irritable bowel syndrome have been mixed, some people use acupuncture to help relax muscle spasms and improve bowel function.

Guar gum. Partially hydrolyzed guar gum has been shown beneficial in animal and human studies, but its potential role in treating IBS needs more study.

Artichoke leaf extract. One small study suggests the extract may help relieve IBS symptoms and is more tolerable than some other treatments.

May help and likely won't hurt

Although research is unclear or mixed on how effective they are, several therapies that are commonly used for IBS, and which carry relatively low risk, are hypnosis, relaxation therapy and yoga.

Dealing with stress may prevent IBS

Finding ways to deal with stress can be extremely helpful in preventing or alleviating symptoms of IBS. These include:

Counseling. Sometimes, a health care professional such as a psychologist or psychiatrist can help you learn how to reduce stress.

Biofeedback. This stress-reduction technique helps you reduce muscle tension and slow your heart rate with the feedback of a machine.

Regular exercise, yoga, massage or meditation. You can take classes in yoga and meditation or practice the therapies at home using books or tapes.

Progressive relaxation exercises. Start by tightening the muscles in your feet, then concentrate on slowly letting all of the tension go. Next, tighten and relax your calves. Continue until the muscles in your body, including those in your eyes and scalp, are completely relaxed.

Deep breathing. Most adults breathe from their chests. But you become calmer when you breathe from your diaphragm, the muscle that separates your chest from your abdomen. When you inhale, allow your belly to expand with air; when you exhale, your belly contracts.

Hypnosis. A trained professional teaches you how to relax and then guides you as you imagine your intestinal muscles becoming smooth and calm.

Memory problems

Increasing evidence suggests that the phrase "Use it or lose it" may indeed apply to your body's most powerful organ — your brain. And that intellectual stimulation — especially, perhaps, in your later years — is key to keeping your brain alive and well.

Will your mental ability change as you age? Research indicates that the answer is yes, it probably will. Like physical performance, mental performance generally tends to decline with age.

It's important to remember, too, that many factors besides age affect mental ability. Depression and chronic stress are the most common. Both can cause difficulty with short-term memory, decreased focus and concentration, and impaired decision-making ability. Both are also treatable.

Memory does depend on the individual, but most people generally can develop valuable habits to help offset age-related memory changes. Mentally stimulating activities such as reading regularly, taking classes, learning new skills and engaging in active conversations with friends may lead to preservation of mental abilities with age.

Conventional Strategies

Are there things that you can do later in life to preserve your mental capacities? Research says, absolutely, yes. Older adults can learn just as well as can younger adults, and it's possible to increase brain cell connections, regardless of your age. Other lifestyle measures also have been shown to benefit mental functioning, such as physical activity, limiting alcohol use and managing stress.

And even if research hasn't outlined all of the ins and outs of the human intellect, keeping your brain active and engaged in the world around you makes for an interesting life — and who can resist that possibility? Being engaged with life pays.

Here are practical strategies to help you keep your brain in shape:

Use reminders and keep organized

In today's world, information comes at you constantly from multiple sources. You need to find a way to get beyond the information overload. To get organized, create a way to track each type of information. List appointments in a personal calendar. Create to-do lists for unscheduled tasks. Maintain a personal file with names, addresses and phone numbers. Even a simple list above the phone will do. A wide variety of tools are available to help you organize, maintain and remember data — ranging from simple paper records to sophisticated computer software.

Create routines, rituals and cues

Keep frequently used items in the same place, whether at work or at home. Have a designated spot to put your car or house keys after each time you use them. Keep the kitchen utensils that you use every day in the same location.

Rituals also can help. Complete common tasks in the same order or at the same time. Also set up cues. For example, place packages to mail close to the front door so that you don't forget them.

Experiment with memory techniques

Experiment with the following to see what works for you:

Make associations. One way to remember something new is to associate it with something else that you already know. You did this as a child when you learned to recognize Italy on a world map by remembering that the country is shaped like a boot.

Choose your memories. Sometimes it's necessary to remind yourself of what's truly important. When meeting many new people at the same time, for example, focus on remembering just a handful of key names. When reading a book or article, give it a quick skim to decide what facts or ideas are important to remember, then let go of the rest.

Repeat, rehash and revisit. Exercise your memory by retrieving key information. Repeat essential facts — names, dates, numbers — several times when you first try to learn them.

Don't be afraid of challenges

Test your limits. Take classes — learn yoga or Pilates or take a philosophy course. Switch careers or start a new one. Take up a new hobby.

Take care of yourself

Caring for your body will help your mind. Staying physically active, getting enough sleep, limiting your alcohol intake and managing your stress levels all contribute to keeping your brain at its optimum functioning level.

Complementary & Alternative Treatment

There are a variety of nonconventional approaches to memory preservation, many of which need further study. Among them are:

Ginkgo. Some research indicates that ginkgo may enhance memory. It generally appears safe when consumed in recommended quantities, but it can increase the risk of bleeding. Talk to your doctor before using ginkgo if you're on a blood-thinning medication.

Ginseng. The evidence is mixed on the effectiveness of ginseng for mental performance, including memory enhancement. But risks of trying it appear low, as serious side effects seem rare. However, ginseng may increase the risk of bleeding in people taking anticoagulant medications, and it may lower blood sugar. Use it under a doctor's supervision.

Omega-3 fatty acids. Limited evidence suggests that consuming higher amounts of omega-3 fatty acids (fish oil) may be associated with improved cognitive function and reduced risk of dementia later in life.

ARA and DHA. A small Japanese study suggests the fatty acids arachidonic acid (ARA) and docosahexaenoic acid (DHA) may improve memory problems associated with aging.

Huperzine A. A couple of studies suggest huperzine A may improve memory and cognitive function in people with dementia.

Phosphatidylserine. The supplement may improve attention and memory in people with cognitive deterioration.

Vitamin B-12. Poor memory can be caused by a vitamin B-12 deficiency (pernicious anemia). In this instance, supplementing with vitamin B-12 may help. There's no evidence that vitamin B-12 supplements are of benefit in treating people with normal memory or with Alzheimer's disease.

May help and likely won't hurt

Several therapies fall into this category, including music therapy, acupuncture, art therapy, coenzyme Q10, guided imagery and pet therapy.

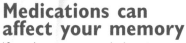

Medications can affect your memory

If you're concerned about your ability to remember, ask your doctor about the side effects of medications you're taking.

Some medications have side effects that can interfere with memory. When you talk to your doctor, mention everything you're taking, including vitamins, minerals, over-the-counter drugs and herbal supplements.

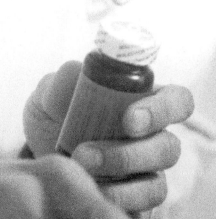

Menopause symptoms

Although your mother or grandmother may have used "the change" to refer to menopause, it isn't a single event. Instead, it's a transition that can start in your 30s or 40s and last into your 50s or even 60s. You may begin to experience signs and symptoms of menopause well before your periods stop permanently. Once you haven't had a period for 12 consecutive months, you've reached menopause.

Menopause is a natural biological process. Although it's associated with hormonal, physical and psychosocial changes in your life, menopause isn't the end of your youth or of your sexuality. Several generations ago, few women lived beyond menopause. Today, you may spend as much as half of your life after menopause.

In recent decades, hormone therapy (HT) has been widely used to relieve the signs and symptoms of menopause and — doctors thought — to prevent diseases associated with aging. However, new long-term evidence has demonstrated that HT may actually increase your risk of serious health conditions, such as heart disease, breast cancer and stroke.

Estrogen therapy is still a safe, short-term option for some women, but numerous other therapies also are available to help you manage menopausal symptoms and stay healthy during this important phase of your life.

Conventional Treatment

Treatments for menopause focus on relieving bothersome signs and symptoms and on preventing or lessening chronic conditions that may occur with aging. Conventional treatments include:

Medications

Hormone therapy. Hormone therapy — estrogen or a combination of estrogen and progestin — remains the most effective treatment option for menopausal symptoms such as hot flashes and vaginal discomfort. However, certain risks exist with long-term hormone therapy, including a slightly increased risk of heart disease, stroke and breast cancer. Depending on your personal and family medical history, your doctor may recommend hormone therapy in the lowest dose needed to provide symptom relief.

Low-dose antidepressants. Venlafaxine (Effexor), an antidepressant related to a class of drugs called selective serotonin reuptake inhibitors (SSRIs), may decrease hot flashes by up to 60 percent. Other SSRIs may also be helpful. Side effects may include nausea, dizziness or sexual dysfunction.

Gabapentin (Neurontin). This drug is commonly used to treat seizures and chronic pain, but it has also been shown to significantly reduce hot flashes. Side effects may include drowsiness, dizziness, nausea and swelling.

Clonidine (Catapres, others). Clonidine, a pill or patch typically used to treat high blood pressure, may reduce the frequency of hot flashes, but side effects such as dizziness, drowsiness, dry mouth and constipation are common.

Bisphosphonates. Doctors may recommend these nonhormonal medications, such as alendronate (Fosamax) and risedronate (Actonel), to reduce bone loss and risk of fractures. In women, these medications have replaced estrogen as the main treatment for osteoporosis. Side effects may include nausea, abdominal pain and irritation of the esophagus.

Selective estrogen receptor modulators (SERMs). SERMs are a group of drugs that includes raloxifene (Evista). Raloxifene mimics estrogen's beneficial effects on bone density in postmenopausal women, without some of the risks associated with estrogen. Hot flashes are a common side effect of raloxifene. You shouldn't use this drug if you have a history of blood clots.

Vaginal estrogen. To relieve vaginal dryness, estrogen can be used in vaginal tablet, ring or cream form. This treatment releases a small amount of estrogen locally to vaginal tissue, and can help relieve vaginal dryness, discomfort with intercourse and some urinary symptoms. Before deciding on any form of treatment, talk with your doctor about your options and the risks and benefits involved with each.

Self-care

Cool hot flashes. If you're experiencing hot flashes, get regular exercise and try to pinpoint what triggers your hot flashes. Triggers may include hot beverages, spicy foods, alcohol, hot weather and even a warm room.

Decrease vaginal discomfort. For vaginal dryness or discomfort with intercourse, use over-the-counter water-based vaginal lubricants (Astroglide, K-Y Jelly), moisturizers (Replens, Vagisil) or vaginal estrogen. Staying sexually active also helps.

Optimize your sleep. If you have trouble sleeping, avoid caffeinated beverages and don't exercise right before bedtime.

Complementary & Alternative Treatment

Many therapies have been promoted as aids in managing the symptoms of menopause. Some complementary and alternative approaches include:

Isoflavones. Soy is a common source of isoflavones — plant-derived compounds that have weak estrogen-like effects. These compounds may help with hot flashes. Study results regarding their safety and effectiveness are mixed — some indicate that isoflavones may increase breast cancer growth, others that they may inhibit it. If you've had breast cancer, talk to your doctor before taking isoflavone pills, such as soy.

Black cohosh. This herb is used for treating hot flashes and other menopausal symptoms. The North American Menopause Society supports short-term use of black cohosh for relieving menopausal symptoms because it seems to have a low risk of side effects when used for up to six months. How it works and the effects of long-term use are uncertain.

Vitamin E. Vitamin E may provide relief from mild hot flashes for some women, when ingested in doses up to 400 international units (IU) daily. However, more recent reports have questioned its safety for cardiovascular health when taken in higher doses over a long term.

Ginseng. Ginseng may help improve mood and sleep problems, but it doesn't help with hot flashes.

Flaxseed. A couple of small studies indicate that flaxseed may help improve menopausal symptoms.

Other therapies. Techniques that focus on relaxation (deep breathing, guided imagery, yoga) don't directly target the hormonal fluctuations of menopause, but they may help you cope with mood swings, stress and sleep disturbances.

Conflicting or unclear evidence

A number of other alternative therapies are used for menopausal symptoms, including red clover, dong quai, chasteberry, evening primrose oil and wild yam (natural progesterone cream). Scientific evidence as to their effectiveness and long-term safety is lacking.

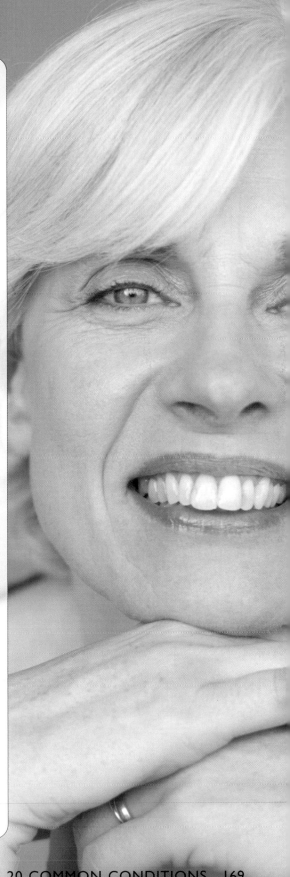

Overweight

Do you weigh more than you should? If so, you're like the two-thirds of American adults who are overweight. About one in three American adults is considered to be obese. And childhood obesity is at an all-time high.

Obesity is more than a cosmetic concern. Being seriously overweight puts you at greater risk of developing high blood pressure and many other serious health risks that may ultimately be life-threatening.

The good news is that even a modest weight loss — reducing your weight by about 5 percent to 10 percent — can bring health improvements. This can often be done through diet and exercise modifications. If that isn't enough, other forms of treatment, including medications and surgery may help.

Talking to your doctor openly and honestly about your weight is one of the best things you can do for your health. The more your weight increases, the more health problems you may face. In addition to high blood pressure, added weight puts you at risk of high blood cholesterol, diabetes and arthritis. All of these conditions may improve if you're able to lose weight.

When it comes to weight loss, there's no shortage of advice. But what you should be looking for is something that works for a lifetime — not a "quick fix."

Conventional Treatment

The safest and most effective way to lose weight is to eat a healthier diet, exercise and change unhealthy behaviors. But this requires a lifelong commitment. In some cases, you may need additional help, perhaps in the form of prescription medications or surgery.

Lifestyle changes

Diet. Calories you eat but don't use up are stored as fat on your body. Consuming fewer calories is an important factor for successful weight loss. The number of calories you need to maintain weight each day depends on several factors, including your age and activity level. Ask your doctor to help you determine your calorie goals to lose weight. He or she may recommend that you also work with a dietitian or a reputable weight-loss program.

Exercise. Changing your diet will help you consume fewer calories, but increasing your physical activity will help you burn calories you've stored up. In the long run, regular exercise is a key component to maintaining weight loss. Use aerobic exercise to burn body fat and strength training to build lean muscle tissue.

Behavior. Last but not least, it's important to change your approach to eating and activity. Long-term weight control relies on lifestyle changes that last. To be successful, you may need to change entrenched habits and beliefs that have hindered weight loss for you in the past. A therapist or a professionally led support group can often be helpful.

Medications

Sibutramine (Meridia). This medication changes your brain chemistry, making you feel full more quickly. Studies have shown that after a year, Meridia users lost an average of about 10 pounds more than did people simply following a low-calorie diet and taking an inactive pill (placebo). Side effects can include increased blood pressure, headache, dry mouth, constipation and insomnia.

Orlistat (Xenical). Orlistat inhibits the absorption of fat in your intestines. Unabsorbed fat is eliminated in the stool. Side effects include oily and frequent bowel movements, but these improve with decreased fat intake. Average weight loss with Xenical is modest, similar to Meridia. Because Xenical blocks absorption of some nutrients, your doctor may recommend that you also take a multivitamin.

Surgery

When appropriate, weight-loss surgery can result in dramatic improvements in weight and health. In the first year or two, most people lose up to 50 percent of their excess weight. Generally, those who follow

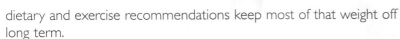

dietary and exercise recommendations keep most of that weight off long term.

Most procedures create a small pouch at the top of your stomach that can hold only about an ounce or two of food, though this can later expand to several ounces. After the operation, you can eat only small portions of food at a time without feeling nausea or discomfort. A variation on this procedure adds a bypass around part of your small intestine, where most of the calories from foods that you eat are absorbed. It reduces what you can eat, and it reduces the calories your body absorbs.

Complementary & Alternative Treatment

Many herbal supplements have been touted as weight-loss aids. Unfortunately, there doesn't seem to be any specific supplement that works well, and some may have potentially dangerous side effects.

Small, preliminary studies suggest the following supplements may have weight-loss potential, but the evidence is still far from conclusive.

Pyruvate. Pyruvate, in the form of pyruvic acid, is found in the body during digestion. As a supplement, it seems safe and may help with weight loss. Taking more than 5 grams a day may cause bloating, gas and diarrhea.

Conjugated linoleic acid (CLA). Animal studies suggest that this compound may reduce body fat and increase muscle. Occasional side effects may include nausea and indigestion.

Calcium. There's some evidence that increasing calcium consumption from dairy products such as yogurt may increase weight reduction. Calcium supplements don't appear to produce the same effect.

Green tea. Green tea may help burn calories and boost metabolism. If you like the taste, it's unlikely to harm you. It does contain a small amount of caffeine, so drinking it in great quantities may hinder sleep.

Omega-3 fatty acids. There's some evidence that the fatty acids in fish oil can improve weight loss.

Chromium. Taking chromium picolinate supplements might produce modest weight loss, but not all studies have shown this benefit.

Not recommended

Some weight-loss supplements are best left on the shelf, including ephedra, bitter orange and country mallow (heartleaf). These supplements can cause potentially dangerous cardiovascular problems. Ephedra supplements have been banned from the marketplace. The ban has been challenged but to date it's still in place. Ephedra may still be sold legally as a tea. Ephedra products also can be found on the Internet.

For more information on herbal weight-loss products, see page 50.

Are you a fidgeter?

Some people have a built-in mechanism for keeping weight off through their everyday movements. Studies show that people who fidget burn extra calories. Fidgeting appears to help them control their weight, even when they overeat.

In one of the most detailed and data-rich studies on obesity ever performed, Mayo Clinic researchers found that people who move more during the day — including fidgeting, tapping their toes, wiggling and changing posture — are less likely to gain weight than are people who move less. Researchers labeled this factor non-exercise activity thermogenesis, or NEAT.

The study provides an optimistic message, even if you're not a fidgeter. Every calorie you burn by moving counts. Even browsing in a store takes twice as much energy as sitting in a chair. If you move more each day, you'll tend to stay leaner than if you sit still.

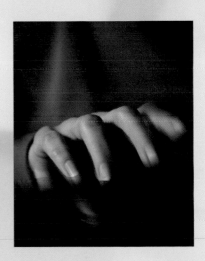

Premenstrual syndrome (PMS)

Mood swings, tender breasts, a swollen abdomen, food cravings, fatigue, irritability and depression. If you experience some or all of these symptoms in the days before your monthly period, you may have premenstrual syndrome (PMS).

An estimated three of every four menstruating women experience some form of premenstrual syndrome. These problems are more likely to trouble women between their late 20s and early 40s, and they tend to recur in a predictable pattern. Yet the physical and emotional changes you experience with premenstrual syndrome may be more or less intense with each menstrual cycle.

Still, you don't have to let such problems control your life. In recent years, much has been learned about premenstrual syndrome. Treatments and lifestyle adjustments can help you reduce or manage the signs and symptoms of premenstrual syndrome.

If you've tried managing your premenstrual syndrome with lifestyle changes, but with little or no success, and signs and symptoms of PMS are seriously affecting your health and daily activities, see your doctor.

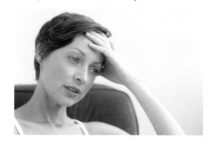

Conventional Treatment

Your doctor may prescribe one or more medications for premenstrual syndrome. The success of medications in relieving symptoms varies from one woman to the next. There are also self-care measures that you can try to ease your symptoms.

Medications

Nonsteroidal anti-inflammatory drugs (NSAIDs). Taken before or at the onset of your period, NSAIDs such as ibuprofen (Advil, Motrin, others) or naproxen sodium (Aleve) can ease cramping and breast discomfort common to PMS.

Oral contraceptives. Oral contraceptives stop ovulation and stabilize hormonal swings, thereby helping to relieve PMS symptoms.

Antidepressants. Selective serotonin reuptake inhibitors (SSRIs), which include fluoxetine (Prozac, Sarafem), paroxetine (Paxil) and sertraline (Zoloft), have been successful in reducing symptoms such as fatigue, food cravings and sleep problems. These drugs are generally taken daily. But for some women with PMS, use of antidepressants may be limited to the two weeks before menstruation begins.

Medroxyprogesterone acetate (Depo-Provera). For severe PMS, this injection can be used to temporarily stop ovulation. However, Depo-Provera may cause an increase in some signs and symptoms of PMS, such as increased appetite, weight gain, headache and depressed mood.

Self-care

Modify your diet. The following may reduce symptoms:
- Eat smaller, more frequent meals each day to reduce bloating and the sensation of fullness.
- Limit salt and salty foods to reduce bloating and fluid retention.
- Choose foods high in complex carbohydrates, such as fruits, vegetables and whole grains.
- Choose foods rich in calcium. If you can't tolerate dairy products or aren't getting adequate calcium in your diet, you may need a daily calcium supplement.
- Take a daily multivitamin supplement.
- Avoid caffeine and alcohol.

Incorporate exercise into your regular routine. Go for a brisk walk, cycle, swim or do another aerobic activity most days of the week. Regular exercise can alleviate symptoms such as fatigue and a depressed mood.

Reduce stress. Get plenty of sleep. For those days when you don't feel well, keep your schedule simple.

Record your symptoms for a few months. Identify the triggers and timing of your symptoms so that you can intervene to help lessen them.

Complementary & Alternative Treatment

Here are some of the more common complementary products and remedies used to soothe the symptoms of premenstrual syndrome:

Calcium. Consuming 1,000 milligrams (mg) of dietary and supplemental calcium daily, such as chewable calcium carbonate (Tums, Rolaids, others), may reduce the physical and psychological symptoms of PMS. Regular use of calcium carbonate also reduces your risk of osteoporosis.

Research also suggests that a high intake of calcium and vitamin D may reduce a woman's risk of PMS.

Magnesium. Taking 400 mg of supplemental magnesium daily may help to reduce fluid retention, breast tenderness and bloating in women with premenstrual syndrome.

Vitamin B-6. A daily dose of 50 to 100 mg of vitamin B-6 may help some women with troublesome PMS symptoms.

Vitamin E. This vitamin, taken in 400 international units (IU) daily, may ease PMS symptoms, including cramps and breast tenderness. However, recent reports have questioned its safety when taken in higher doses over a long term.

Black cohosh. This herb, native to North America, is often used to treat menopausal symptoms and may reduce premenstrual cramps. How it helps is uncertain. Some studies suggest it has estrogen-like properties; others contradict this. Side effects may include headaches and stomach discomfort. Clinical trials of black cohosh have lasted for only six months or less, so longer term side effects are unknown. It's recommended that you don't take it for more than six months unless your doctor approves. Pregnant women should avoid black cohosh, as it may induce miscarriage.

Chasteberry. The fruit of the chaste tree, called the chasteberry, has been used for centuries to treat women's hormone-related problems. Research suggests that chasteberry may reduce breast pain, swelling, constipation, irritability, depressed mood, anger and headache. In general, it seems to be well tolerated with only mild side effects. However, chasteberry isn't considered safe if you're pregnant or breast-feeding.

Dong quai. The Chinese herb dong quai, a type of wild celery, has been used for thousands of years to treat PMS. It's thought to relieve symptoms by easing internal organ spasms. Chinese research also suggests that it may stimulate the production of red blood cells, increasing energy and reducing fatigue. Dong quai may increase your sensitivity to sunlight and sunburn, especially if you're fair skinned. It's not recommended for women who are pregnant or breast-feeding.

Ginkgo. There's some evidence that ginkgo may reduce breast tenderness associated with PMS.

Relaxation therapy. Practice progressive muscle relaxation or deep-breathing exercises to help reduce headaches, anxiety or insomnia.

Premenstrual dysphoric disorder: A severe form of PMS

Up to 8 percent of menstruating women have PMDD — a severe, sometimes disabling form of premenstrual syndrome.

PMDD is distinguished from PMS by the severity of its symptoms and its impact on relationships and daily activities. Symptoms may include persistent sadness, anxiety, fatigue, feelings of being overwhelmed, flu-like symptoms and changes in sleeping and appetite patterns.

What causes PMDD isn't clear. Frequently, women with PMDD also have major depression, but not always.

A doctor may diagnose premenstrual dysphoric disorder based on its pattern of symptoms. Your doctor may recommend that you keep a diary to record the type, severity, duration and timing of your symptoms. This information may help your doctor diagnose PMDD and determine the most appropriate treatment for you.

Antidepressants known as selective serotonin reuptake inhibitors (SSRIs) are often the first line of therapy for PMDD. Other therapies used to treat premenstrual syndrome, including chasteberry, may also be helpful for PMDD.

Sexual problems

Although you may feel as if you're the only one who experiences difficulties with your sexual life, you're far from being alone. Many people — both men and women — experience sexual problems at some point in their lives. However, such concerns tend to become more common with age.

For men, erectile dysfunction (impotence) is a common problem. Patterns of erectile dysfunction may range from an occasional inability to obtain a full erection to an inability to maintain an erection throughout intercourse to an inability to achieve an erection at all.

For women, sexual dysfunction implies persistent or recurrent problems encountered in one or more of the stages of sexual response. This may include low or absent desire for sex, difficulty in achieving or maintaining sexual arousal, inability to achieve orgasm and painful sexual intercourse.

When sexual problems prove to be persistent and distressing, they can interfere with a person's self-image and his or her relationships. Although sexual problems are often multifaceted, they are treatable. And whereas sexual concerns were once considered a taboo subject, doctors and their patients are realizing that frank communication and better understanding of the nature of the problems are important steps toward sexual health.

Conventional Treatment

For both men and women, treatment often requires first addressing an underlying medical condition or adjusting medications that have sexual side effects. Counseling or psychotherapy can be useful not only for the person experiencing difficulties but also for his or her partner.

For men

Oral medications. These include sildenafil (Viagra), tadalafil (Cialis) and vardenafil (Levitra). They work by enhancing the effects of nitric oxide, a chemical messenger that relaxes smooth muscles in the penis. This increases blood flow and allows an erection to occur in response to sexual stimulation. Don't combine these medications with nitrate drugs, such as nitroglycerin. Together, they can cause dizziness, low blood pressure and loss of consciousness.

Prostaglandin E (alprostadil). Alprostadil is a synthetic version of the hormone prostaglandin E, which helps enhance blood flow needed for an erection. The medication can be injected with a fine needle at the base of the penis or as a tiny suppository inserted into the tip of the penis.

Hormone therapy. For the small number of men who have testosterone deficiency, testosterone replacement therapy may be an option.

Vacuum devices. This treatment involves using a hand pump to pull blood into the penis and create an erection. A tension ring placed around the base of the penis maintains the erection during intercourse.

Vascular surgery. Surgery is usually reserved to correct blood flow in men who've experienced an injury to the penis or pelvic area.

Penile implants. This treatment involves surgically placing an inflatable or semirigid device into the two sides of the penis, which you manipulate at will. This treatment isn't usually recommended until other methods have been considered.

For women

Pelvic floor exercises (Kegels). These exercises strengthen the muscles involved in pleasurable sexual sensations and may help with arousal and orgasm difficulties. To do the exercises, tighten your pelvic muscles as if you're stopping your stream of urine. Hold for a count of five, relax and repeat several times a day.

Estrogen therapy. Localized estrogen therapy in the form of a vaginal cream, gel or tablet can help with sexual changes due to menopause. Estrogen may help improve the tone and elasticity of vaginal tissues, increase vaginal blood flow and enhance lubrication.

Progestin therapy. Some studies suggest that progestin hormonal therapy, in combination with estrogen, may lead to improvements in desire and arousal. More research is needed.

Testosterone therapy. Testosterone is important for sexual function in women as well as men, although at a much lower level. But its use for sexual dysfunction is controversial.

Complementary & Alternative Treatment

Although there are a number of proposed alternative remedies for sexual dysfunction, scientific evidence as to their safety and effectiveness is limited. These remedies include:

Acupuncture. A few small, preliminary studies suggest that acupuncture may possibly help improve erectile dysfunction. Acupuncture uses ultrafine needles inserted at strategic points on your body to improve your body's flow of vital energy. Acupuncture risks are generally low.

DHEA. In its natural form, dehydroepiandrosterone (DHEA) is the raw material from which male and female sex hormones are generated. DHEA levels in the body begin to decline after age 30. A few clinical trials suggest that, in its synthetic form, DHEA may possibly increase libido in premenopausal women and improve erectile dysfunction in men, but more study is needed. Acne is a common side effect.

Ginkgo. This herbal extract may help erectile dysfunction by improving blood flow to the penis. It may also improve sexual side effects of antidepressants in both men and women. Ginkgo may increase your risk of bleeding, so talk to your doctor before taking it if you're also on blood-thinning medications.

L-arginine. L-arginine is a protein that occurs naturally in the body. In its supplement form, it may help erectile dysfunction by enhancing the effects of nitric oxide, not unlike the action of Viagra and similar medications. Side effects may include nausea, abdominal cramps and diarrhea, especially at higher doses. Don't take L-arginine with Viagra.

Be cautious

Yohimbe bark extract. Derived from the yohimbe tree of western Africa, this bark extract has been traditionally used as an aphrodisiac and mild hallucinogen, but little research has been done on it. Its close cousin, yohimbine hydrochloride (Yocon) — a standardized prescription drug — is used for treating sexual side effects of antidepressants, female sexual dysfunction and erectile dysfunction. Yohimbe bark extract may contain yohimbine but levels vary, so it's difficult to know what you're getting. High doses can be dangerous. All forms may increase heart rate and raise blood pressure. Therefore, it's best to avoid this product.

'Herbal viagras.' Sildenafil (Viagra) is a prescription medication used to treat erectile dysfunction. Many herbal products are touted as "herbal viagras," but they're not the same as Viagra. For more information on these products, see page 63.

Coping with ED

Whether the cause is physical or psychological, or a combination of both, erectile dysfunction (ED) can become a source of mental and emotional stress for a man — and his partner.

If you experience erectile dysfunction only on occasion, try not to assume that you have a permanent problem or to expect it to happen again during your next sexual encounter. Don't view one episode as a lasting comment on your health, virility or masculinity.

In addition, if you experience occasional or persistent erectile dysfunction, remember your sexual partner. Your partner may see your inability to have an erection as a sign of diminished sexual desire. Your reassurance that this is not the case can be helpful.

To appropriately treat erectile dysfunction and strengthen your relationship with your partner, try to communicate openly and honestly about your condition. Couples may also want to seek counseling to confront any concerns they may have about erectile dysfunction and to learn how to discuss their feelings. Try to maintain this communication throughout the diagnosis and treatment process.

Treatment is often more successful if couples work together as a team.

Stress and anxiety

Modern life is full of pressures, fears and frustration. In other words, it's stressful. Racing against deadlines, sitting in traffic, arguing with your spouse — all of these situations make your body react as if you were facing a physical threat.

This reaction — called the "fight-or-flight response" — gave early humans the energy to fight aggressors or run from predators. It helped the species survive. Today, instead of protecting you, stress may — if constantly activated — make you more vulnerable to health problems.

It's normal to feel anxious or worried at times — everyone does. But if you often feel anxious without reason and your worries disrupt your daily life, you may have what's called generalized anxiety disorder (GAD). This condition causes excessive or unrealistic anxiety and worry about life circumstances, usually without a readily identifiable cause.

Fortunately, there's help for chronic stress and anxiety. Treatment ranges from learning new coping skills to medications to professional counseling or therapy. Several complementary and alternative therapies may also prove helpful in easing your emotional and physical burden.

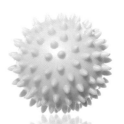

Conventional Treatment

If you're under continuous stress that appears to have no endpoint in sight, you may be able to help yourself by implementing some key changes in your life. Professional counseling also can help. A buildup of stress can lead to generalized anxiety disorder, in which case a combination of medications and psychotherapy is often recommended.

Self-care

There are three fundamental ways in which to manage stress: By changing your environment so that daily demands aren't so high, by learning how to better cope with the demands in your environment, or by doing both.

Techniques that can help you manage stress include identifying and addressing those problems you can change, letting go of stressors beyond your control, taking good care of yourself, maintaining a healthy diet, exercising and finding time for relaxation, and relying on certain people to help you through the rough spots.

Medications

Anti-anxiety drugs. Benzodiazepines are sedatives that often ease anxiety within 30 to 90 minutes. Because they can be habit-forming, your doctor may prescribe them for only a short time to help you get through a particularly anxious period. Side effects include unsteadiness, drowsiness, reduced muscle coordination and problems with balance. Higher doses and long-term use can cause memory problems.

Antidepressants. These drugs influence the activity of certain brain chemicals (neurotransmitters) to help nerve cells (neurons) in your brain send and receive messages. Antidepressants usually begin to work within two weeks, but it may take up to eight weeks before you notice their full effects. You may need to try more than one to find which drug works best for you.

Psychotherapy

A common form of psychotherapy used to treat anxiety is cognitive behavior therapy. During treatment sessions, a therapist helps you identify distorted thoughts and beliefs that trigger psychological stress, fear or depression. You learn to replace negative thoughts with more positive, realistic perceptions, and you learn ways to view and cope with life events differently.

Complementary & Alternative Treatment

Various forms of complementary and alternative therapies are used to treat stress and anxiety. The success of these treatments often depends

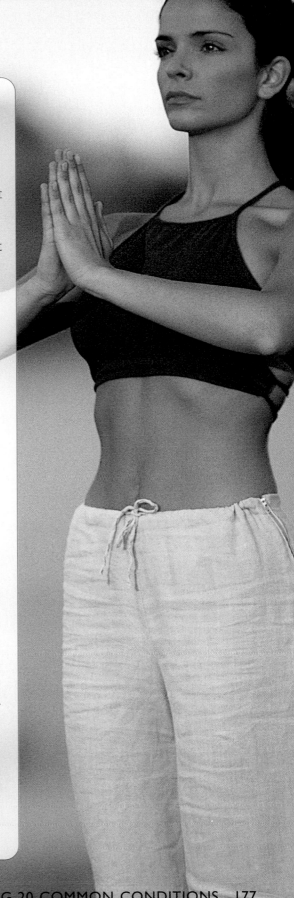

on each individual's response. With the exception of some herbal therapies, most are relatively safe and have few side effects.

Herbal therapy. Kava, St. John's wort, passionflower and valerian are some of the most common herbal extracts used for anxiety. Research shows kava to be effective in soothing tension and agitation, but reports of severe liver damage have been associated with its use, therefore it's not recommended. Kava has been banned from sale in some countries, and other countries are considering similar action.

St. John's wort has mostly been studied for treatment of depression but there's some evidence that it may also help relieve anxiety. St. John's wort can interact with many different medications and supplements, so be sure to talk with your doctor before taking this supplement.

Passionflower and valerian — often taken in the form of bedtime tea — appear to have mild sedative and tranquilizing properties with few side effects.

Biofeedback. For this technique, a practitioner measures your body's physiological response to stress or anxiety, which is displayed to you as auditory or visual signals. By increasing your awareness of your body's responses, you attempt to counter the signals with relaxation methods.

Relaxation therapy. Relaxation therapy encompasses numerous techniques ranging from paced respiration and deep breathing to meditation and progressive muscle relaxation. Most involve repetition of a single word, phrase or muscular activity and promote "emptying" your mind of external thoughts and stressors.

Massage. A number of studies indicate that massage can help reduce stress and anxiety symptoms.

Aromatherapy. Aromatherapy is the science of using oils from various plants to treat illness and promote health. The oils are often vaporized and inhaled or used as massage oils. It's believed that compounds in the oils activate certain parts of your brain, releasing different brain chemicals that may have a relaxing effect.

Art and music therapy. Art therapy involves the use of drawing, painting, clay or sculpture to allow expression and organization of your inner thoughts and emotions when talking about them is difficult. The creation of art itself, or interpretation of an art piece, is thought to be therapeutic. Playing of music — even during medical procedures — has also been shown to produce relaxing and calming effects.

Yoga. When practiced regularly, yoga may help reduce daily stress and anxiety. Kundalini yoga, a type of yoga that's been studied specifically for anxiety disorder, combines poses and breathing techniques with chanting and meditation.

Acupuncture. A study conducted at Mayo Clinic found that acupuncture helped reduce anxiety symptoms associated with fibromyalgia.

Vaginal yeast infections

For many women, the itching, burning vaginal sensations and white, lumpy discharge that accompany vaginal yeast infections are all too familiar. And they usually produce the feeling of "Oh, no, not again."

Yeast infections are common — an estimated three out of four women will have a yeast infection in their lifetimes, and about half of women have two or more infections.

Yeast infections occur when certain internal or external factors change the normal environment of your vagina and trigger an overgrowth of a microscopic fungus — the most common being a fungus called *Candida albicans* (*C. albicans*). A yeast infection isn't considered a sexually transmitted disease.

Certain medications (antibiotics, steroids), uncontrolled diabetes, and hormonal changes caused by pregnancy or birth control pills can make you more prone to yeast infections. Bubble baths, vaginal contraceptives, damp or tightfitting clothing, and feminine hygiene sprays and deodorants also may increase your susceptibility to infection.

Fortunately, treatment is readily available. Once you've learned to recognize a yeast infection, you can usually treat it with over-the-counter products, with the approval of your doctor.

Conventional Treatment

Yeast infections generally are treated with an antifungal cream or suppository. You should see your doctor if this is your first vaginal infection, you've had more than one kind of vaginal infection, you've had multiple sex partners or a recent new partner, or if your symptoms persist despite treatment. Also see your doctor if you experience a fever or develop a particularly unpleasant vaginal odor. It's possible you have something other than a yeast infection.

Self-care

If you've talked to your doctor and you know that you have a yeast infection, your doctor may recommend going ahead with treatment on your own, taking these steps:

- Use an over-the-counter medication specifically for yeast infections. Options include one-day, three-day or seven-day courses of cream or vaginal suppositories. The active ingredient in these products is clotrimazole (Gyne-Lotrimin), miconazole (Monistat) or tioconazole (Vagistat). Some products also come with an external cream to apply to the labia and opening of the vagina to soothe itching. Follow package directions and complete the entire course of treatment even if you're feeling better right away.
- To ease discomfort until the antifungal medication takes full effect, apply a cold compress, such as a washcloth, to the labial area.

If you experience persistent infections, your doctor may also prescribe for you a single dose of the oral medication fluconazole (Diflucan).

Preventive care

To help prevent vaginal yeast infections, consider the following:

- Don't douche. The vagina doesn't require cleansing other than normal bathing. Repetitive douching disrupts the normal organisms that live in the vagina and can actually increase the risk of vaginal infection. Douching won't clear up a vaginal infection.
- Avoid potential irritants, such as scented tampons or pads.
- Wear cotton underwear and pantyhose with a cotton crotch. Don't wear underwear to bed. Yeast thrives in moist environments.
- Change out of wet swimsuits and damp clothing as soon as possible.

Complementary & Alternative Treatment

Some popular home remedies for treating or preventing vaginal yeast infections include a cream made from tea tree oil, vaginal suppositories made with garlic or boric acid, and douching with vinegar. Anecdotally, some women report success with these home remedies. However, well-designed controlled trials are needed to investigate their safety and effectiveness before any reliable recommendations can be made.

Yogurt. *Lactobacillus acidophilus* (*L. acidophilus*) is a type of beneficial bacteria normally found in the vagina. One study found that vaginal suppositories containing *L. acidophilus* improved symptoms of vaginal yeast infections. However, other studies of oral preparations of *L. acidophilus* found little benefit. Another option is to eat yogurt that contains active lactobacillus cultures. This is a healthy habit that may have the added bonus of reducing recurrent vaginal yeast infections. Evidence as to the effectiveness of eating yogurt to fend off such infections is inconclusive, but there's no risk in giving it a try.

Echinacea. One study found taking echinacea supplements in combination with a topical antifungal cream was effective in preventing recurrent vaginal yeast infections.

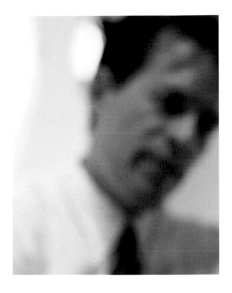

Can men get yeast infections?

A man can get a yeast infection from sexual contact with a woman who has a yeast infection. However, not every man exposed to a yeast infection will get one. Men are at increased risk of such an infection if they have diabetes or are uncircumcised.

Signs and symptoms of male yeast infection include:
- Itching or burning at the head of the penis
- Red rash on the penis

A male yeast infection is usually a relatively minor problem that can be easily treated with the same antifungal creams or ointments used to treat female yeast infections.

If the rash doesn't go away after about a week or it recurs frequently, see your doctor.

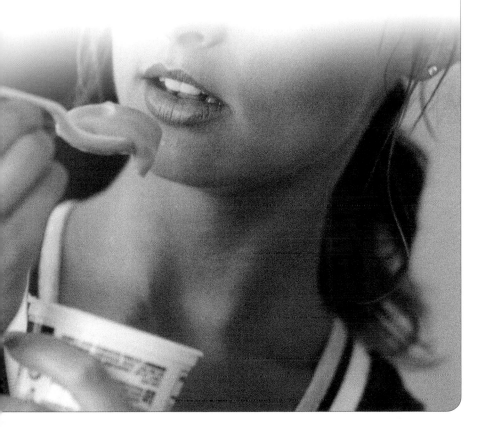

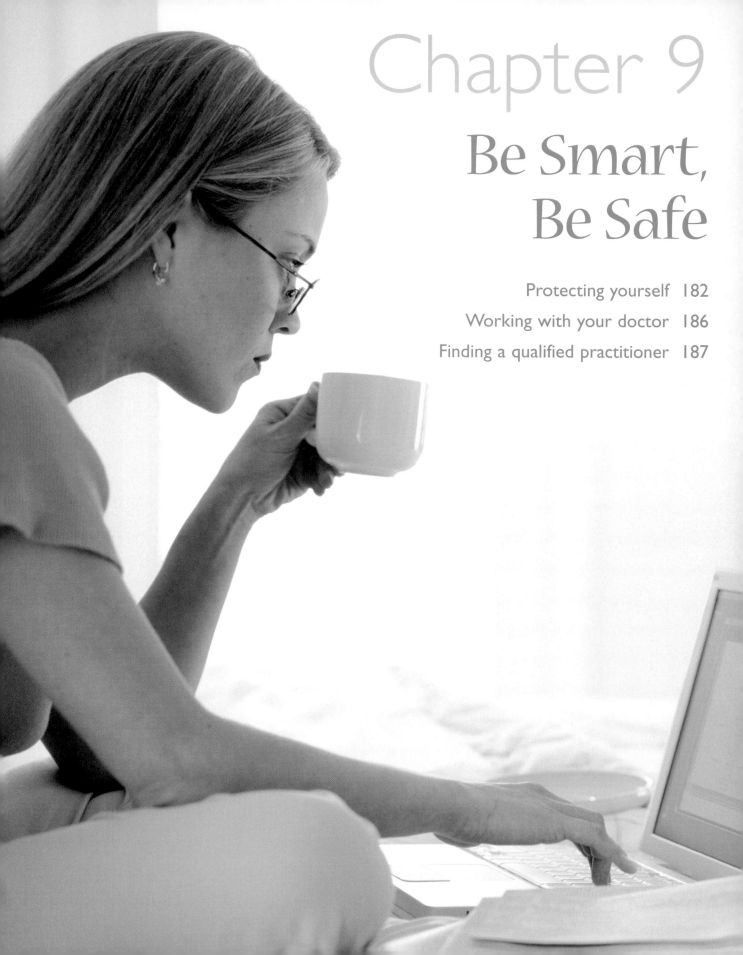

Chapter 9

Be Smart, Be Safe

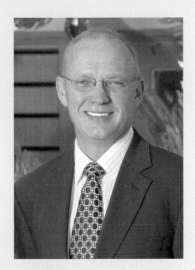

Larry Bergstrom, M.D.
Complementary and
Integrative Medicine Program

" *Unfortunately, when it comes to complementary and alternative therapies, the information available about many products is based on benefits to the company advertising the product rather than on benefits to the user.* "

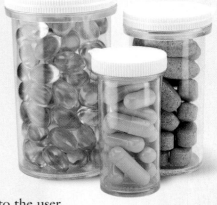

"It's natural!" That's the answer I get frequently from my patients when I inquire why they're taking an herbal supplement.

More than ever before, people are involved and interested in their health care. They seek out information about the latest in treatments and practices reported to be beneficial to their health and happiness. Unfortunately, when it comes to complementary and alternative therapies, the information available about many products is based on benefits to the company advertising the product rather than on benefits to the user.

I'm also finding that a number of my patients use multiple products, in the belief that they're helping themselves. And they trust that the products are safe. Alternative and complementary products and practices may offer benefits when it comes to your health. But some of them also pose risks — serious risks. Many supplements come from plants whose ingredients are powerful agents. St John's wort, for example, interacts with many prescription medications and can lead to serious health risks for individuals who combine the supplement with a medication. In addition, some natural plant substances used in supplements are actually poisonous — the poison serving as protection against the plant being eaten!

The option to pick and choose among treatments — alternative, complementary and conventional — provides great opportunities to maintain health and happiness. But it also makes the complicated world of health care even more so. Take a careful look at your options. Make sure the therapy you're considering will do you more good than harm — consider its safety as well as its effectiveness. A safe practice is one that does no harm when it's used as intended.

Finally, to reduce potential risks, you need to be up front with your doctor. Your health is your doctor's No. 1 priority, but he or she can't help protect you if you don't provide honest answers. Many patients I encounter neglect to report all of the health products and supplements they're using, either because they don't consider them to be relevant or they're uncertain how I may react to their using the products. Your doctor needs to know about everything you're taking — prescription or nonprescription — including natural products.

Remember, your doctor has the same goal that you do — to help you live a healthy and long life.

Protecting yourself

It's becoming increasingly evident that complementary and alternative medicine can play a role in better health. But it's important to remember that there are some important differences between conventional treatments and complementary and alternative therapies.

If you decide to use complementary and alternative treatments, protecting your health — and your wallet — requires you to do two things.

First, learn about these treatments. Find out what they are and what benefits their practitioners claim they provide. Second, take responsibility for your own well-being. Before choosing a treatment, evaluate the benefits and risks.

5 steps to follow

When considering any product or practice, do your homework.
1. **Gather information.** The Internet offers an ideal way to keep up with the latest on complementary and alternative treatments. If you don't have Internet access at home or work, contact public libraries. But beware — the Internet is also a great source of misinformation.
2. **Evaluate the providers.** After gathering information about a treatment, you may decide to find a practitioner who offers it. Choosing a name from the classified section of the phone book is

risky if you have no other information about the provider. Check your state government listings for agencies that regulate and license health providers. These agencies may list names of practitioners in your area and offer a way to check credentials.

Many official-sounding organizations may not be reputable. Talk with your doctor or another trusted health care professional to get advice.

Talk to people who've received the treatment you're considering and ask about their experience with specific providers. Before you agree to treatment, call the provider to schedule an informational interview.

There are risks and side effects with many types of treatment. With any treatment that you consider, determine if the benefits outweigh the risks.
3. **Consider the cost.** Many complementary and alternative approaches aren't covered by health insurance. Find out exactly how much the treatment will cost you. Whenever possible, get the amount in writing before you begin treatment.
4. **Check your attitude.** When it comes to complementary and alternative medicine, steer a middle course

between uncritical acceptance and outright rejection. Learn to be open-minded and skeptical at the same time. Stay open to various treatments, but evaluate them carefully. In addition, remember that the field is changing: What's alternative today could well be accepted — or discredited — tomorrow.
5. **Opt for complementary over alternative.** The best use of alternative therapies is to complement rather than replace conventional medical care.

You can use complementary treatments to maintain good health and to relieve some symptoms. But continue to rely on conventional medicine to diagnose a problem and treat the sources of disease.

Be sure to seek conventional treatment if you have a sudden, severe or life-threatening health problem.

Also, remember that lifestyle choices make a difference. Most medical practitioners — conventional, complementary and alternative — will tell you that good nutrition, exercise, not smoking, stress management and safety practices are keys to a long life and good health.

Dietary supplements: Not your typical pills

Walk into the vitamin aisle of any pharmacy, discount or grocery store, and you'll find them — herbal remedies such as echinacea, ginkgo and garlic.

Herbs, vitamins and minerals are all considered dietary supplements by the Food and Drug Administration (FDA). Though often thought of as less risky than prescription medications, dietary supplements aren't subject to the same quality controls as drugs.

Limited regulation

In 1994, Congress passed the Dietary Supplement Health and Education Act (DSHEA). This law limits the FDA's control over products labeled dietary supplements. The DSHEA states that manufacturers don't have to prove to the FDA that a product is safe or effective before it goes on the market.

As a result, in the United States herbs can be marketed with limited regulation. Vendors can make health claims about products based on their own review and interpretation of studies — without FDA authorization. However, the FDA can pull a product off the market if it's proved dangerous.

Safe use

If you use dietary supplements:

- **Follow directions.** Similar to nonprescription and prescription drugs, herbal products have active ingredients that can affect how your body functions. Don't exceed the recommended dosages. Some herbs can be harmful if you take too much or take them for too long.

- **Tell your doctor what you're taking.** Some herbs may interfere with the effectiveness of prescription or over-the-counter drugs or have other harmful effects.

- **Keep track of what you take.** Take one type of supplement at a time to determine if it's effective. Make a note of what you take, how much and how it affects you. Do you experience any side effects, such as drowsiness, sleeplessness, headache or nausea?

- **Read the label and look for a seal of approval.** Quality and strength can vary greatly by brand. Look for a seal of approval from an independent verification program, such as the U.S. Pharmacopeia's "USP Dietary Supplement Verified" mark, indicating that the supplements meet certain standards of quality.

- **Avoid supplements if you're pregnant or breast-feeding.** They could harm your baby. Take them only if your doctor approves.

- **Be cautious about products manufactured or purchased outside the United States.** Some European herbs, such as German herbs, are well regulated and standardized. But toxic ingredients (including lead and mercury) and prescription drugs (such as prednisone) have been found in herbal supplements manufactured elsewhere, particularly China, India and Mexico.

- **Avoid potentially dangerous herbs altogether.** These include a variety of herbs such as chaparral, ephedra (ma-huang) and kava. Overdoses of any of these herbs can be fatal. Though some of these are "banned," they're still available over the Internet and by other means.

Case in point

Here's one example to illustrate how you don't always know what you're getting when it comes to dietary supplements.

The consumer safety organization ConsumerLab.com conducted a study of garlic supplements. It found only six of 14 products studied contained the amount of garlic expected, based on product labels. One product didn't contain any of a key garlic compound, and another had less than 1 percent of the expected amount.

Clearly, some dietary supplements are of high quality, but it can be difficult, if not impossible, to distinguish them from the rip-offs, without laboratory testing.

The best approach — when possible — is to choose whole foods over pills, so you know what you're getting. If you're seeking the benefits of garlic, add garlic to your food. If you're after the benefits of vitamin C, eat an orange. Whole foods also provide numerous other nutrients that supplements don't.

Is it helping?

Once you begin using a particular complementary or alternative therapy, make sure to periodically assess if the product or practice is working.

You likely won't see changes overnight, but after a period of four to six weeks you should be able to determine if it's helping.

Ask yourself the following questions:

- **Why did I decide to use this particular product or therapy?** Was it to reduce pain, reduce stress or bolster your immune system?
- **Am I noticing a difference?** Has the pain lessened, or your stress level eased? Do you feel better? Are you getting fewer colds?
- **Am I bothered by side effects?** Are you experiencing unwanted effects from the therapy, such as headache, nausea or muscle pain? Do the benefits outweigh the side effects?
- **What's my goal?** Is the product or therapy working well enough to help you achieve your goal?

If you're not seeing the results you hoped for, talk with your doctor. It may be that you're not using the therapy correctly, or that you're not taking the right amount.

Or it could be that the product or practice simply doesn't work for you. Why waste your money or time on something that isn't helpful? You and your doctor may want to consider your alternatives and try a different approach.

Sounds too good to be true? Maybe it is.

The Food and Drug Administration and the National Council Against Health Fraud recommend that you watch for the following claims or practices. These are often warning signs of potentially fraudulent dietary supplements or other so-called "natural" treatments:

- The advertisements or promotional materials include words such as *breakthrough, magical* or *new discovery*. If the product were in fact a cure, it would be widely reported in the media and your doctor would recommend it.
- Promotional materials include pseudo-medical jargon such as *detoxify, purify* or *energize*. Such claims are difficult to define and measure.
- The manufacturer claims that the product can treat a wide range of symptoms, or cure or prevent a number of diseases. No single product can do this.
- The product is supposedly backed by scientific studies, but references aren't provided, are limited or are out of date.
- The product's promotional materials mention no negative side effects, only benefits.
- The manufacturer of the product accuses the government or medical profession of suppressing important information about the product's benefits. There is no reason for the government or medical profession to withhold information that could help people.

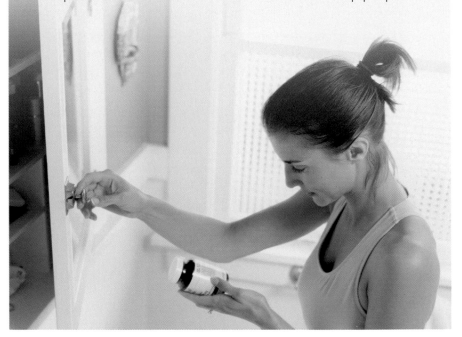

When medicines and herbs don't mix

Modern medicine is just beginning to understand individual herbs and other dietary supplements.

One question that researchers want to learn more about is what happens when herbs are mixed with prescription or nonprescription medications.

For the time being, think twice before mixing any herb with a prescription or nonprescription drug. Certain herbs have been recognized as having a high risk of interactions. Following are some examples.

Herbs of concern

Don't mix medications with these popular herbs, unless you have your doctor's approval:

- Echinacea

- Feverfew

- Garlic

- Ginger

- Ginkgo

- Ginseng

- Kava

- St. John's wort

Medications of concern

Some medications have a narrow therapeutic window. That is, significant problems can develop if the level is too low or too high. An example is the anti-coagulant medication warfarin (Coumadin). If the level is too low, dangerous blood clotting can occur. If the level is too high, dangerous bleeding can occur.

If you take the following medications, it's especially important that you not take any supplement without talking with your doctor. There may be other medications that don't interact with certain supplements.

- The cardiac drug digoxin

- Medications to control heart arrhythmias (anti-arrhythmics)

- Medications to prevent organ rejection

- Medications to control seizures

- Warfarin

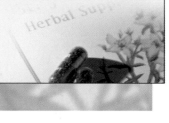

66 *Think twice before mixing any herb with a prescription or nonprescription drug.* 99

Play it safe during pregnancy

If you're pregnant or are trying to become pregnant it's very important that you discuss alternative therapies with your doctor. Many therapies — especially herbal and other dietary supplements — aren't recommended for women who are pregnant or planning to become pregnant because they can harm the baby.

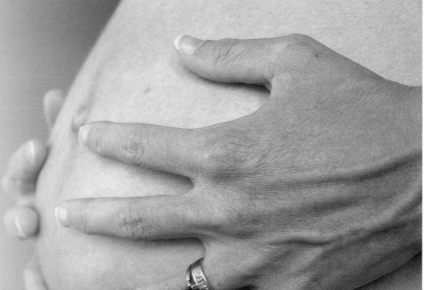

Working with your doctor

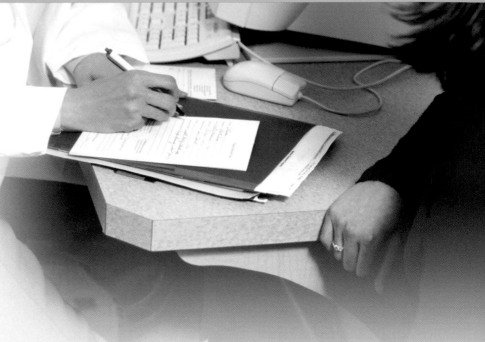

You may be a little gun-shy when it comes to talking with your doctor about complementary or alternative therapies that you're using, or are considering using.

Perhaps you're worried that your doctor will criticize you or tell you to stop using the treatment. If the therapy isn't dangerous, this shouldn't be the case. Most doctors are well aware that unconventional products and practices are highly popular, and they want to help their patients use the therapies safely.

Surveys also show that because people often consider therapies such as herbs "natural," they don't feel they're worth discussing with their doctor. Remember, natural doesn't mean safe. Tell your doctor about everything that you take.

Act sooner, rather than later

It's best to talk with your doctor before taking any dietary supplement. Also inform your doctor about other therapies you may be considering, such as meditation or acupuncture.

Why? Your doctor is there to help you. He or she can:

- Determine if the treatment has any potentially dangerous side effects
- Help you determine the appropriate dosage
- Provide advice on which therapies are most appropri-

ate for you, given your overall health status

- Inform you if a product you're considering taking may interact with a medication you currently use
- Put you in touch with someone who can perform a particular therapy or who can teach you how to do it

It's important that you answer your doctor's questions accurately. Honest communication between you and your doctor helps your doctor to better monitor your health and assess potential health risks.

Understand the unease

When it comes to dietary supplements, don't be surprised if

your doctor may be cautious about endorsing or embracing some of them. This is often because relatively few controlled studies have been done on dietary supplements.

Understandably, the more evidence there is to support a particular product or practice, the more comfortable doctors feel in recommending it.

However, a growing number of doctors are working to better understand herbal and other supplemental therapies so that they can help you make informed decisions about your health care.

If your doctor isn't comfortable discussing dietary supplements with you, ask for a referral to a pharmacist or specialist who is knowledgeable in this area.

Finding a qualified practitioner

When selecting an individual who practices complementary or alternative medicine, it's important to do your homework and then evaluate your options. Before making an appointment, make sure that you have plenty of information about the provider you're considering.

Where to look

To find a qualified practitioner, you might try checking with:

State regulators

Check your state government listings for agencies that regulate and license health care providers. These agencies may list practitioners in your area and offer a way to check credentials.

National associations

National associations and their local affiliates can usually provide you with the names of certified practitioners in your area. To find the addresses and phone numbers of these associations, visit your local library or use the Internet. Be careful — official-sounding organizations aren't always reputable. Talk with your doctor or another trusted health care professional for advice.

Friends and family

If you know someone who's received the same treatment you're considering, he or she can offer advice. Ask about his or her experiences with a specific provider.

Points to keep in mind

The National Center for Complementary and Alternative Medicine (NCCAM) suggests you follow these steps when deciding on a practitioner:

- Speak with your primary health care provider or someone you believe to be knowledgeable about the therapy you're interested in. Ask for a recommendation.

- Make a list of practitioners and gather information about each. Ask questions about their credentials and practice. What licenses or certifications do they have?

- Find out what the treatment will cost. Whenever possible, get it in writing. Many alternative approaches aren't covered by health insurance.

- After you select a practitioner, make a list of questions to ask at your first visit. Decide if the potential benefits outweigh the risks.

- Come to the first visit prepared to answer questions about your health history, as well as any prescription medicines, vitamins and other supplements you may take.

- Assess your first visit and decide if the practitioner is right for you and the treatment plan is reasonable and acceptable.

Our wish for you

We hope this book has filled you with enthusiasm to try something new — whether it be meditating for the first time or attending a yoga course. By making a commitment to care for yourself — mind, body and spirit — you can reap the benefits of improved health and wellness in the years to come.

Health care in the United States may be facing significant challenges in the coming years. But those same challenges can create unique opportunities for each of us to play a more active role in promoting our own health and wellness.

It's our hope that you will return to this book and use it as a guide as you explore new ways of nourishing your whole self.

We also hope this book encourages you to create partnerships with all of your health care providers. Be patient with your doctors and give them a chance to learn along with you. Many of the subjects in this book are fairly commonplace, but many others are still quite foreign to doctors who trained several years ago.

Best wishes for a life of health and wellness!

The Editors

Additional Resources

Organizations

Acupuncture and Oriental Medicine Alliance

P.O. Box 738
Gig Harbor, WA 98335
253-238-8133
www.aomalliance.org

American Academy of Medical Acupuncture

4929 Wilshire Blvd., Suite 428
Los Angeles, CA 90010
323-937-5514
www.medicalacupuncture.org

American Academy of Osteopathy

3500 DePauw Blvd., Suite 1080
Indianapolis, IN 46268
317-879-1881
www.academyofosteopathy.org

American Association of Naturopathic Physicians

4435 Wisconsin Ave. N.W., Suite 403
Washington, DC 20016
866-538-2267
www.naturopathic.org

American Association of Oriental Medicine

P.O. Box 162340
Sacramento, CA 95816
866-455-7999
www.aaom.org

American Botanical Council

P.O. Box 144345
Austin, TX 78714
800-373-7105
www.herbalgram.org

American Chiropractic Association

1701 Clarendon Blvd.
Arlington, VA 22209
703-276-8800
www.amerchiro.org

American Holistic Medical Association

P.O. Box 2016
Edmonds, WA 98020
425-967-0737
www.holisticmedicine.org

American Massage Therapy Association

500 Davis St., Suite 900
Evanston, IL 60201
877-905-2700
www.amtamassage.org

American Osteopathic Association

142 E. Ontario St.
Chicago, IL 60611
800-621-1773
www.osteopathic.org

American Society of Clinical Hypnosis

140 N. Bloomingdale Road
Bloomingdale, IL 60108
630-980-4740
www.asch.net

Association for Applied Psychophysiology & Biofeedback

10200 W. 44th Ave., Suite 304
Wheat Ridge, CO 80033
800-477-8892
www.aapb.org

ConsumerLab.com, LLC*

333 Mamaroneck Ave.
White Plains, NY 10605
914-722-9149
www.consumerlab.com

Healing Touch International

445 Union Blvd., Suite 105
Lakewood, CO 80228
303-989-7982
www.healingtouchinternational.org

MayoClinic.com

www.MayoClinic.com

National Association for Holistic Aromatherapy

3327 W. Indian Trail Road, PMB 144
Spokane, WA 99208
509-325-3419
www.naha.org

National Center for Complementary and Alternative Medicine

NCCAM Clearinghouse
P.O. Box 7923
Gaithersburg, MD 20898
888-644-6226
www.nccam.nih.gov

* Subscription fee required for access to information

National Center for Homeopathy

801 N. Fairfax St., Suite 306
Alexandria, VA 22314
703-548-7790
www.homeopathic.org

Office of Cancer Complementary and Alternative Medicine

National Cancer Institute, NIH
6116 Executive Blvd., Suite 609, MSC 8339
Bethesda, MD 20892
703-548-7790
www.cancer.gov/cam

Databases

Natural Medicines Comprehensive Database*

www.naturaldatabaseconsumer.com

Natural Standard*

www.naturalstandard.com

Index